PEDIATRIC BEHAVIORAL MEDICINE

Edited by
Ben J. Williams
John P. Foreyt
G. Ken Goodrick

PRAEGER

PRAEGER SPECIAL STUDIES • PRAEGER SCIENTIFIC

Library of Congress Cataloging in Publication Data

Main entry under title:

Pediatric behavioral medicine.

    Bibliography: p.
    Includes indexes.
    1. Pediatrics—Psychological aspects. 2. Sick child-
ren—Psychology. 3. Behavior therapy. I. Williams,
Ben J., 1939-   II. Foreyt, John Paul III. Goodrick, G. Ken. [DNLM: 1. Behavior therapy—in infancy
and childhood. WS 350.6 W721p]
RJ47.5.P33   618.92′001′9   81-5875
ISBN 0-03-059599-1   AACR2

Published and Distributed by the
Praeger Publishers Division
(ISBN Prefix 0-275)
of Greenwood Press, Inc.,
Westport, Connecticut

Published in 1981 by Praeger Publishers
CBS Educational and Professional Publishing
A Division of CBS, Inc.
521 Fifth Avenue, New York, New York 10175 U.S.A.

© 1981 by Praeger Publishers

123456789 145 987654321

Printed in the United States of America

ACKNOWLEDGMENTS

The editors wish to acknowledge the contribution of Dianne Robbins in manuscript preparation. A special thanks is given to the staff of Texas Medical Center Library, Geanene Fenske, Penny Worley, and Gail Hannigan, for their assistance.

CONTENTS

LIST OF TABLES AND FIGURES

LIST OF ABBREVIATIONS AND ACRONYMS

APA	American Psychological Association
ASDC	American Society of Dentistry for Children
CNS	central nervous system
CS	conditioned stimulus
MMPI	Minnesota Multiphasic Personality Inventory
UCS	unconditioned stimulus

1

INTRODUCTION

PEDIATRIC BEHAVIORAL MEDICINE

Over the last ten years there has been increasing recognition that psychological and behavioral factors play an important role in what used to be considered traditional pediatric problems. A large, multifaceted literature has evolved concerning the treatment of psychoneurotic, developmental, psychosomatic, and chronic physical disorders in children, with techniques derived from social-learning principles. These behaviorally based therapies are being applied to a wide variety of problem behaviors in the natural settings of home and school, and in hospitals and long-term care facilities.

The behavioral approach of the 1980s is not limited to the simple stimulus-response models associated with animal research. It has been expanded from the analysis of antecedent cues and consequent social responses to include private events. The cognitive ecology of Michael Mahoney (1974) and the cognitive behavior therapy of Donald Meichenbaum (1977) have paved the way for examination of how internalized language, imagery, and affect influence subsequent behavior. Albert Bandura's (1976) work has given us a perspective on how more complex behaviors are learned vicariously through observation and modeling. Behaviorally oriented therapists now have a number of techniques with which to research and manage many childhood disorders that in the past were not treated effectively.

The Yale Conference on Behavioral Medicine has been particularly helpful for uniting a diverse group of pediatric (and nonpediatric) behavioral and biomedical specialists by defining goals and making recommendations for the emerging field. Schwartz and Weiss (1978), in the first issue of the *Journal of Behavioral Medicine*, elaborated the four conclusions that grew out of the conference. The first defined the specialty:

> Behavioral medicine is the field concerned with the development of behavioral science knowledge and techniques relevant to the understanding of physical health and illness and the application of this knowledge and these techniques to prevention, diagnosis, treatment and rehabilitation. Psychosis, neurosis, and substance abuse are included only insofar as they contribute to physical disorders as an end point. (p. 7)

The second conclusion attempted to specify the content and subareas composing it. The third recognized the existence of a major body of scientific research on behavioral medicine already in existence, as well as a number of specialized journals that represent the field. The last conclusion recommended the forming of a society of behavioral medicine. This recommendation was achieved at the 1978 meeting of the Association for Advancement of Behavior Therapy (AABT) in Chicago. The 1979 AABT convention held in San Francisco was preceded by the first annual meeting of the society.

The field of pediatric behavioral medicine, as it appears now, will be highly interdisciplinary and not a reflection of the special interests of either psychologists or their medical colleagues. It will be research-oriented, with treatment methods flowing from data generated by scientist-practitioners who treat various disorders. It will emphasize applied behavior analysis and will require the use of objectively verifiable and replicable treatment strategies. Perhaps most important of all, pediatric behavioral medicine will take a preventive approach, in agreement with national health-care priorities, to reduce the incidence rates of chronic diseases.

As behavioral techniques have proceeded from sole reliance on the systematic analysis of antecedent and consequent events to the analysis of cognitive and affective states, so in the future analyses must eventually extend to the social system in which individuals live. The behaviorally oriented therapist and researcher must encourage thoughtful and thorough examination of all of our therapeutic and educational ecologies, as well as the general lifestyles of children and their families.

In order to clarify how these techniques and procedures can be used, the following systems model for pediatric behavioral medicine is presented, followed by a review of the techniques used in behavior therapy. A section is then included on how parents and other professionals can be trained in the use of these techniques. A protocol for use of these techniques describes the general procedures to be used in pediatric behavioral medicine from referral to follow-up.

SYSTEMS MODEL FOR PEDIATRIC BEHAVIORAL MEDICINE

When a child has a health problem, the parents will likely consult the services of a pediatrician. If their child's behavior is undesirable, they may go to a child psychologist or other specialist. However, "health" problems satisfactorily treated using only medical techniques, and "behavioral" problems satisfactorily treated using only behavioral techniques represent the ends of a continuum of health-behavior problems that require both medical and behavioral treatment; hence behavioral medicine. In Western cultures health and behavior, or mind and body, have traditionally been dichotomized. This dichotomy is reflected in the traditional separation of health and psychological services. Within this dichotomy, there has been a tendency to think of health or behavioral problems as having a single cause such as a virus or a personality disorder, which is inside the child. More recently, health and psychological providers have recognized the need to integrate their disciplines, since most illnesses have a psychological component, and a large number of childhood behavior problems directly or indirectly affect health. The problems children have are no longer seen as caused solely by a disease entity or psychological problem, but are viewed as manifestations of a larger system of interactions including the children's physical and social environment. Figure 1.1 depicts a systems model for pediatric behavioral medicine. A particular problem may involve only a few elements of this model. However, if a path exists from the child to symptoms or behaviors, to consequences, and back to the child in terms of reinforcement, the path represents the sufficient conditions for development of a chronic problem. Intervention requires the modification of the subsystem represented by this path.

This model can be best understood through the use of a hypothetical example. A child may develop a skin irritation through an exogenous agent such as a burn or abrasion. The initial problem is tissue damage. The associated pain may be viewed as punishing any behavior that would interfere with healing. Most injury-consequences subsystems naturally result in feedback loops that affect behavior in a way that optimizes healing processes. However, this is not always true. The skin injury may begin to itch. The child scratches. The scratching behavior exacerbates the skin condition, leading to more itching. This subsystem may get progressively worse or stabilize in a condition of moderate neurodermatitis. In addition to the skin condition and the scratching behavior, emotional behavior may appear in reaction to the pain or inflamed tissue. These become the consequences of the subsystem for the parents.

A normal response by the parents would be to inspect the condition, apply salve, and instruct the child not to scratch. The attention may have a reinforcing effect on the problem behavior. The salve may reduce the itching. The instructions not to scratch may or may not be effective depending upon

FIGURE 1.1. Systems model for pediatric behavioral medicine

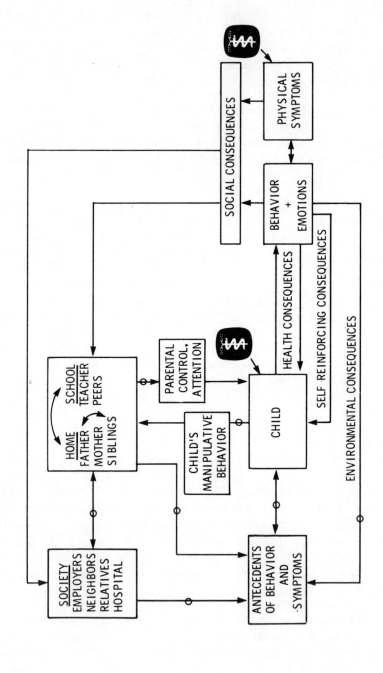

the self-control of the child. If the condition persists, then the parents and perhaps a teacher and school nurse will be brought into the subsystem. The relationship of parents to society is shown as part of the system, since a majority of parents who demonstrate an inability to intervene effectively in their child's pathological subsystems are having difficulty in their social subsystem (for example, in employment, marriage, relations with friends) (Wahler, Berland, & Coe, 1979).

For the pediatrician, there are two places indicated in Figure 1.1 for medical intervention. Medical treatment may be applied to the child that affects the physiological problem, or treatment may be applied that gives symptomatic relief. Such intervention may not bring lasting relief, since it touches only a part of the total system. For the behavioral psychologist, there are many potential places in the system to intervene, depending upon how many components of the model are ultimately involved in the maintenance of the child's problem. If the family appears healthy, intervention in the smaller subsystem of the child might involve having the parents alter the reinforcing consequences of the problem behavior by punishing it or by withholding attention. They may also change the antecedent conditions that lead to problem behaviors. If modification of the child subsystem fails, the larger family system may need help. If the child seems to get attention only when the problem behavior occurs, the parents could be taught to provide more noncontingent attention. If parents are unable to apply systematically a behavioral prescription because of marital problems or problems related to their employment, then therapy is indicated for these problems at a total system level.

The systems model presented should be useful for all persons who treat children's problems. By applying this model to any particular problem, one can determine at what level intervention is necessary. The model should also be a useful teaching device to help explain the complex interactive nature of the system and the rationale for treatment to parents and health professionals.

REVIEW OF BEHAVIORAL TECHNIQUES

Behavioral medicine has as its base the experimental studies of learning and conditioning of Pavlov, Skinner, Wolpe, and others. These behavioral underpinnings emphasize the observable relationships among measurable activities, antecedent stimuli, and subsequent environmental events. Once a problem is identified, one may attempt to accelerate, decelerate, or otherwise affect the topography of a set of behaviors by altering the antecedent conditions, the behavior itself, or the environmental consequences of the behavior. Antecedent stimuli are those events that have been demonstrated either through measurement or observation to regularly precede, in time, the occurrence of the maladaptive behavior under scrutiny. Frequently, the antecedent events serve as cues for the behavior to occur. A mother cooking may serve as the antecedent stimulus for a child's manipulatory behavior related to an eating problem. The behavior may include a temper tantrum, which the child has learned will make the mother provide desired food. Many maladaptive behaviors, such as temper tantrums, may be maintained by the parent unwisely placating the child to avoid the unpleasant experience of hearing it scream. Excessive attention and reassurance to a child about to undergo some dental procedure may serve only to provide the antecedent conditions for the development of a dental phobia.

The article by Shorkey and Taylor (1973) entitled "Management of maladaptive behavior of a severely burned child," in the dermatological chapter, illustrates how clear discrimination between the antecedent stimuli associated with painful treatment of burns and the antecedent stimuli with nurturant care led to the ultimate recovery of a 17-month old child.

Contingency management typically involves training parents, teachers, or professionals in principles of reinforcement. These change agents are taught to "catch the child being good," that is, to reinforce acceptable, prosocial behaviors and to avoid inadvertent reinforcement of unacceptable and undesirable behaviors. Training may take the form of instruction in simple reinforcement, use of one of the numerous behavioral manuals such as Patterson's *Families* (1971a), clinical supervision and modeling via observation or video tape, or instruction in a token economy program. Neisworth and Moore (1972), in the chapter on respiration, demonstrate how parents can reduce chronic asthma through the careful reinforcement of adaptive behavior.

Behavioral shaping or successive approximation is a technique used in conjunction with contingency management to build more complex behavioral repertories from simple reinforced behaviors. Ulan, Juris, and Dornback (1974), in the chapter on vision, describe the use of parent-monitored reinforcement and successive approximation in influencing an amblyopic child to wear an eye patch.

Most studies on the behavioral treatment of common childhood problems involve the use of contingency management and successive approximation. Though many of these are case studies, an excellent experimental literature has evolved, primarily from studies published in the *Journal of Applied Behavior Analysis*. Taken together, the studies on the manipulation of antecedent and consequent events accounted for most of the literature until recently. Of late, studies have begun to look more closely at the actual behavior. The works of Bandura (1969), Mahoney (1974), and Meichenbaum (1977) have encouraged researchers to study not only the cognitive, imaginal, and affective events ongoing within the child but also the role of modeling in the acquisition of more complex social behaviors.

Modeling, behavior rehearsal, and social skills training are being used to teach children who are deficient in interpersonal skills. Adelson and Goldfried (1970), in their article in the dental chapter, illustrate how modeling can be used with preschool children to avoid the development of dental phobias. Assertive training is used with over- and underaggressive children to teach them appropriate social responding. Bär and Kuypers (1973), in the article, "Behavioral therapy in dermatological practice," describe the use of assertive training in the treatment of chronic blushing. An increased emphasis on the analysis and manipulation of covert events in the near future can be expected.

Though the operant approach has proved useful in dealing with child behavioral problems, perhaps due to the fact that children are under the reinforcement control of their parents and teachers, relaxation training and desensitization are also increasingly being used in disorders that have a learned anxiety base. Bär and Kuypers (1973), in their previously cited article, illustrate the use of these techniques with a number of dermatological disorders. Ince (1976), in "The use of relaxation training and a conditioned stimulus in the elimination of epileptic seizures in a child: A case study," used systematic desensitization to decrease anxiety associated with recurrent seizures in a 12-year-old epileptic boy. Azrin and his colleagues (Azrin, Sneed, & Foxx, 1974; Azrin & Nunn, 1973, 1974) in the treatment of enuresis, stuttering, and tics, demonstrate a synthesis of clinical treatment and experimental rigor. Their studies are multifaceted, dealing with a succession of techniques carried out with great clinical skill made for maintenance and generalization of treatment to the natural environment.

A summary of all the techniques and how they were used in this collection of studies is shown in Table 1.1.

PROBLEMS AT HOME: TRAINING PARENTS

Since Wahler, Winkel, Peterson, and Morrison (1965) first trained mothers to be therapists to their problem children, the importance of training parents in behavioral techniques has been recognized (for example, Atkeson & Forehand, 1978; Graziano, 1977; Hall, Axelrod, Tyler, Grief, Jones, & Robertson, 1972; Johnson & Katz, 1973; O'Dell, 1974; Patterson, Cobb, & Ray, 1973; Zeilberger, Sampen, & Sloane, 1968). Patterson and Gullion (1971), in their book *Living with Children*, have organized a number of behavioral principles into an excellent instructional manual that can be readily used by psychologists, educators, and others. Following this pioneering work, a variety of other training manuals have been developed (including Becker, 1971; Hall, 1971; Homme & Tosti, 1971; Madsen & Madsen, 1975; Patterson, 1971a).

TABLE 1.1.   Summary of behavioral techniques used in studies

Contingency Management	Disorder	Intervention	Reference
Positive reinforcement			
Social reinforcers	inappropriate behavior during hearing tests	social praise for quiet behavior; social praise for attending to procedure	Garrard & Saxon (1973)
	enuresis	child praised for using toilet appropriately	Azrin, Sneed, & Foxx (1974)
Food	nonverbal child	food rewards for attending	Stark, Rosenbaum, Schwartz, & Wisan (1973)
	obesity	favored foods, money, and activities awarded for appropriate eating	Wheeler & Hess (1976)
Activities	anorexia nervosa	access to physical activity contingent on weight gain	Liebman, Minuchin, & Baker (1974)
	constipation	child gets to play in tub for passing stool	Lal & Lindsley (1968)
Shaping	refusal to wear patch	reinforcement for successively longer periods of wearing patch	Ulan, Juris, & Dornback (1974)
	dental phobia	social praise and token points for gradually increasing cooperative behavior; points exchanged for prize	Drash (1971)

Technique	Disorder	Description	Reference
	eating problem	praise and preferred foods used as rewards for gradually eating solid foods	Palmer, Thompson, & Linschied (1975)
Tokens	nonverbal child	tokens for appropriate verbal responses	Stark, Rosenbaum, Schwartz, & Wisan (1973)
Reinforced incompatible behaviors	stuttering	cessation of speaking and deep breaths during speech	Azrin & Nunn (1974)
	asthma	parents reinforce incompatible behaviors; noncoughing	Neisworth & Moore (1972)
Punishment	eruresis	verbal disapproval for accident; child had to change bed and practice going to bathroom	Azrin, Sneed, & Foxx (1974)
Extinction	asthma	parental attention to symptoms stopped	Neisworth & Moore (1972)
	ccnstipation	mother stops attending to child on toilet	Lal & Lindsley (1968)
	neurodermatitis	parental attention to scratching stopped	Bär & Kuypers (1973)
	eating problem	mother stops paying attention to interfering verbal behavior at mealtime	Palmer, Thompson, & Linscheid (1975)

(continued)

TABLE 1.1, continued

Contingency Management	Disorder	Intervention	Reference
	sleep disturbance	parents stopped paying attention to child's inappropriate behavior at bedtime and increased attention during the day	Wright, Woodcock, & Scott (1970)
	inappropriate behavior during hearing tests	therapist stopped attending to child's screaming	Garrard & Saxon (1973)
Stimulus control			
	seizures	a cue word associated with relaxation used to relax child to avoid seizures	Ince (1976)
	burn management	feeding staff wore distinct costume so that treatment fears would not interfere with eating	Shorkey & Taylor (1973)
	obesity	analysis and change of stimuli associated with eating	Wheeler & Hess (1976)
Modeling			
	dental phobia	use other child as model who received a reward	Adelson & Goldfried (1970)
Relaxation			
	seizures	relaxation training; desensitization to associated anxiety	Ince (1976)
	stuttering	relaxation training to relax while speaking	Azrin & Nunn (1974)

In addition to the parent-training manuals, audio tapes, video tapes, mechanical signaling apparatus, and "bug-in-the-ear" devices have been utilized (Bernal, 1969; Toepfer, Reuter, & Maurer, 1972; O'Leary, O'Leary, & Becker, 1967). The technology of parent training is growing at a phenomenal rate. Teaching parents the basics of behavior change has the possibility of eradicating or at least ameliorating certain behavior problems in their children and, perhaps more important, providing the parents with skills for preventing the occurrence of problems in the future.

The parent-training manuals all point out that most behaviors, adaptive and maladaptive, are maintained by their effect on the natural environment and can be modified by changing the reinforcing consequences provided by the parents. By modifying the social and physical environment so as not to reinforce maladaptive behaviors but to reinforce more healthful behaviors, the parent can correct the child's previously learned undesirable behaviors. For these newly learned adaptive behaviors to be maintained, the pattern of parent-child interaction must be permanently modified.

Parent training varies widely on a number of dimensions, from highly artificial experimental settings to the natural environment (Berkowitz & Graziano, 1972). The most successful studies occur in the child's home and school. Examples of parent training based on respondent techniques are few in number (Clement, 1970; DeLeon & Mandell, 1966; Graziano, 1971; Lovibond, 1964); most of the research has been on the operant model by which parents are taught the use of differential reinforcement, use of time out and other mild punishment techniques, and extinction. While single case studies are numerous, Hanf (1969), Walder, Cohen, Breiter, Warman, Orme-Johnson, and Pavey (1972), and Patterson (1971b) are examples of large-scale intervention programs.

Hanf (1969) described a six-week, two-stage program of 15 half-hour laboratory sessions, utilizing modeling and direct training of mother and child. A "bug-in-the-ear" apparatus and video-taping were used to train mothers to reinforce their children in the laboratory setting. Hanf's program was innovative in his emphasis on generalized interactions, but none of the training occurred in the natural environment.

Walder, et al. (1972) described a 15-week parent-training program designed to build better interactions within the family system. Parents were trained in behavioral analysis and in the application of operant principles to parent-child relations. The program included a contingency contract technique, weekly group meetings to teach and demonstrate the basic principles of behavior theory and technology, and sessions with their family-consultant centering on specific application strategies. Though the Walder et al. (1972) program contained many innovative features and a sound curriculum approach, it provided little data to support the efficacy of the techniques.

Patterson (1971b) reported what perhaps might be one of the best programs to date. Parents were exposed to a ten-to-twelve week training program that required them to master each sequence of the training before proceeding to the next sequence. They were first trained to master *Living with Children* (Patterson & Gullion, 1971), and then taught by the staff how to observe, record, target, and track problem behaviors. They then joined a parents' group in which they were supervised in carrying out behavioral change programs. Patterson has evolved quite an elaborate, comprehensive, and reliable behavior coding procedure that clearly depicts complex social interactions. Utilizing his coding procedure, he has demonstrated generalization across settings, improvement in the behaviors of siblings of problem children, and improvement in parents' descriptions of their children.

The use of parent-training manuals and behavioral training courses is increasing rapidly and will undoubtedly become a major function of behaviorally oriented child psychologists and psychiatrists in the near future. Long-term follow-up data are now needed to assess the effectiveness of this approach to behavioral problems.

PROBLEMS AT SCHOOL: TRAINING TEACHERS

The importance of the academic and informal psychosocial experiences of each child in the classroom cannot be overemphasized. Becker (1973) notes that most of the "innovative" ideas regarding education have been known and used by educators and psychologists for 40 or 50 years. However, in the absence of convincing research and a useful technology for dealing with the learning environment, teachers have had to rely on coercive methods. Excessive attention is paid to disruptive and nonstudy behaviors with little attention to adaptive, study, and social behaviors.

Hart, Reynolds, Baer, Brawley, and Harris (1968) have demonstrated that social reinforcers from adults can strengthen behaviors in children. Baer (1966) concluded that contingent use of adult attention could influence a wide variety of problems, including hyperactivity, dependency, inattentiveness, aggression, and poor language. Subsequent research has seen these techniques applied to almost all social and academic behaviors. An impressive array of studies has been published, principally in the *Journal of Applied Behavior Analysis*, as well as in other behavioral journals, *Behavior Therapy, Journal of Behavior Therapy and Experimental Psychiatry*, and *Behaviour Research and Therapy*.

Madsen, Becker, Thomas, Kosar, and Plager (1968), for example, demonstrated that the more frequently first-grade teachers asked their children to sit down the more frequently the children stood up. This is a clear example of how teacher attention, negative or positive, can function to maintain the exact behavior that the teacher or parents seek to change. Becker (1973) has concluded that 80 to 90 percent of classroom behavior problems can be handled by little more than modifying the teacher's use of attention, that is, use of rule setting, positive reinforcement for adaptive behaviors, and ignoring or "time out from positive reinforcement" for disruptive behaviors.

In an attempt to train teachers, several easily readible, highly interesting, and very practical manuals have been developed. These manuals seek to teach the teacher how to use the basic principles of behavior modification and to show in practical ways how to deal with problem behaviors. Some of the more outstanding manuals include those by Buckley and Walker (1970), Zifferblatt (1970), Homme, Csanyi, Gonzales, and Rechs (1969), and Hewett (1969). Several of the studies included in this volume (for example, Ayllon, Layman & Kandel, 1975) involved the teacher's use of behavioral principles to modify a child's disorder in the school setting.

PEDIATRIC BEHAVIORAL CONSULTATION

Being multidisciplinary in nature, pediatrics is accustomed to consultation from allied health disciplines. However, prospective behavioral consultants face a number of problems when they attempt to enter pediatric settings. In their enthusiasm, some may rush ahead in unselective ways, creating forces of resistance in pediatric care teams. Resistance results either in the eventual demise of the original behavioral goals or in a delay in the consultation. All too often prospective consultants are medically naive, insensitive to systems implications of behavioral consultation, or not prepared to do the work of relationship building necessary for the implementation of behavioral techniques. For therapists who are already employed in an institution where consultation is anticipated, the role is much easier. However, all prospective consultants should familiarize themselves with the pediatric literature associated with the problems under study, as well as with related behavioral techniques that have been applied or might be applied to the problems of concern. Prospective consultants should avail themselves of pediatric clinical conferences that are a regular part of the teaching aspect of hospital settings. Gaining access to these conferences allows them to become known to the medical social system in which they wish to consult, and also to become aware of the clinical realities, the pediatric problems, and the limitations of the health care delivery system. Not only must they consider ways to apply behavioral techniques to particular problems under consideration, but they must perform behavioral analyses of the social system within which they wish to consult.

Consultation in the pediatric setting may be established at the initiative of either the pediatric consultee or the behavior therapist. The invitation to consult usually comes in the form of a request either to present a clinical case or to meet with a group of pediatric personnel. Here the task for behavioral consultants is to gain admittance to a series of regularly occurring meetings to which they may make input. Therapists who wish to establish consultation on their own initiative run a greater risk of rejection than those who are invited to consult. Entry into the system may be gained through a simple request to be allowed to attend a clinical teaching seminar on a regular basis; through offers of case-centered consultation, or in-service training for professional, supervisory, and primary care personnel; or through search and program evaluation. The level of entry into the system determines the initial type of consultation. Therapists may enter as consultants to pediatricians, to assist with research program evaluations or to help with difficult cases. They may also enter the system as consultants to the nursing staff or to supervisory personnel. They may consult regarding the training of nursing personnel or regarding general issues of nursing care delivery. Additionally, they may enter at the level of the primary child care workers whose principal responsibility is to provide 24-hours-a-day treatment to institutionalized children. At any level of entry into the health care system, therapists must have the approval, sanction, and active support of all personnel in the hierarchy. Behavior therapists must resist impulses to begin immediate case-centered consultation but instead should enlist the personnel to teach them the nature of the health care delivery system and the politics, folkways, mores, and perceived needs of the team, as well as the particular management and treatment adherence problems characteristic of their population. They need to look closely at the current management techniques and how the individuals and the treatment unit accommodate to everyday clinical problems.

Though behavioral consultants initially might suggest how personnel are inadvertently reinforcing unacceptable behaviors or attitudes in their young patients and families, they might do better by carefully delineating and pointing out the adaptive functions already existent within the system. Consultants should not suggest reordering of the system, but should seek to improve its quality and efficiency through the use of behavioral methodology. To do this, they must show how to deal more effectively with the day-to-day management problems. They must not only be able to demonstrate an understanding of the dynamics of the system and a sensitivity to the role definitions and feelings of the personnel, but must also provide them with suggestions that improve rather than threaten their jobs. Resistance to change is always a fact of life, even in the face of overwhelming evidence that change is necessary. Because of this resistance to change, consultants must work for slow but carefully planned progress.

It is generally not consultants but rather consultees who determine whether consultation will occur, the extent of its effectiveness, and the general form it will take. Behavioral consultants must engage the pediatric consultees in a process that educates them to the value of their methodology. To avoid rejection, prudent consultants should attempt to adapt their conception of what might be helpful to the consultees' perception of their needs. Consultants who do not have the skills or interest to consult in the manner prescribed by the social system, would do better to exit from the system or serve as facilitators to bring in consultants who can adapt to the perceived needs.

Feedback to personnel at various levels typically functions to create further desire for information and a recognized need for education in behavioral techniques. At that point, consultants may take a case-centered approach in which they will "take over" and treat cases. This strategy frequently backfires because primary care personnel often interpret the consultants' actions as discrediting their own present level of functioning. Rather, behavior therapists might offer case-centered consultation to the primary care workers with the goal of helping them to manage their patients effectively and also offer, if requested, some in-service training in broader aspects of behavioral methodology. If at all possible, training should be offered during regular work hours.

Consultation must be a continuing process of data gathering, assessment of progress, and goal attainment through data analysis. Care must be taken to improve the staff's ability to do their jobs and, at the same time, to avoid overloading them with elaborate data systems that relate more to the research orientation of the consultants than to the orientation of the pediatric health care delivery team. Behavioral consultants must be available at regular hours to consult with personnel on both a case and a systems level basis. Though many of the behavioral medicine problems covered in this book have well-defined procedures for treatment, others will require a research orientation until effective treatment procedures have been developed. The value of data gathering and an experimental orientation must be clearly explained to persons whose primary goal is health care delivery. Once an adequate base of knowledge is established in personnel, and patients are being treated through the use of behaviorally oriented techniques, consultants must then direct themselves toward issues of maintenance and generalization of treatment effects outside the medical environment. They must explore new and more efficient means of applying the behavioral technology to particular medical difficulties. Finally, consultants must also engage health care personnel in a continuing process of training.

With the increasing growth of behavioral medicine, the curriculums of pediatric, child psychiatric, and family practice residents, as well as of other medical and dental specialties, need to include behavioral instruction and supervised practice. It is not enough for medical residents or dental students to have a reading knowledge sufficient to pass their respective board exams: they need supervised experience with these techniques. Just as behavior therapists have developed teaching materials to use with parents and teachers, so they must develop materials and procedures for medical personnel who wish to become familiar with behavioral techniques. Behavioral consultants should pay attention to physicians and resident staffs in fostering their interest in some of the more advanced practical applications of the techniques. Behavior specialists who wish to work or consult in medical settings need to receive continuing training in learning theory and newer behavioral techniques as well as training in the psychological aspects of pediatric problems, information about common pediatric syndromes, and consultation skills particular to the pediatric field.

BASIC PEDIATRIC BEHAVIORAL MEDICINE PROTOCOL

Figure 1.2 is a flow chart showing the stages of treatment from the entry point into the health care system to long-term follow-up. This chart is applicable to any childhood disorder whether it is construed as a medical problem, a behavioral-emotional problem, or a behavioral medicine problem. When medical and behavioral treatments are combined, their effects must be evaluated separately so that a total treatment protocol can be devised that minimizes intrusive or pharmacological medical treatment and results in behavioral treatments that ultimately approximate the behavioral control conditions for normal development. This evaluation is necessarily a long-term process that begins with medical and behavioral diagnoses and ends with long-term follow-up. Each case requires some trial and error to discover optimal combinations of medical and behavioral treatment.

The entry point will be determined primarily by the parents' perception of their child's disorder as either a medical or a behavioral problem. Since parents usually have an ongoing relationship with a pediatrician as a matter of course, the pediatric office is the major entry point. Some health clinics now include both pediatricians and child psychologists (Schroeder, 1979) so that all behavioral-medical aspects of a disorder can be diagnosed and treated. Since many medical and behavioral services are at present not coordinated, the behavioral medicine approach requires interdisciplinary referrals. Unless the disorder is clearly unidisciplinary, careful coordination of treatment effort will be required at each stage.

The diagnostic procedure followed by the pediatrician will be directed towards the exploration of possible underlying organic pathology as a cause of the disorder. Such a procedure is of course mandatory when any child presents apparent physical symptoms. Because of the present health care delivery system, a separate pediatric exam and treatment regimen will usually occur without a behavioral consultation. In many cases the disorder will not have a behavioral component; the medical treatment will be sufficient.

FIGURE 1.2. Basic pediatric behavioral medicine protocol

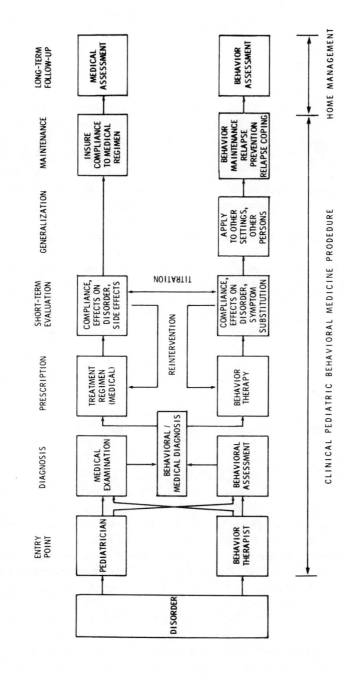

However, getting the family to comply with the treatment regimen may require a behavioral approach. Also, many child disorders that are maintained in whole or in part by behavioral problems get their start from an episode of medical illness.

If the medical treatment ultimately is unsuccessful, or if the problem is originally suspected to have a behavioral etiology, then behavioral assessment is in order. Assessment procedures for behavior therapy of children have been described in detail (McAuley & McAuley, 1977). In behavioral medicine for children the assessment procedure will be much the same, except that the medical symptoms and behavior associated with medical treatment regimens will be included.

In a preliminary interview with parents and child, a clear description of the disorder will be taken. If medical help has been obtained, the procedures associated with treatment become part of the total picture. Any other problems the child or family has should be brought out, since most behavioral disorders of children stem from inappropriate parenting and family discord. For this reason, the therapist should discover how the parents control the child's behavior, whether they use predominantly a positive reinforcement or a punishment approach, and whether they are a highly verbal or nonverbal family. This assessment may indicate family therapy for a more positive and verbal home environment.

The child's social skills and academic performance should be carefully assessed. Since many maladaptive behaviors associated with medical disorders are reinforced by parental attention, the therapist should determine how much the child desires attention and when the parents provide it. Other assessment procedures might include intelligence testing and a neuropsychological battery to check for minimal cerebral and associated neurological dysfunction.

The first week or so of behavioral treatment should always include a detailed baseline measurement of the behavior associated with the disorder and all events surrounding it that may have an effect. Pertinent data to be collected include frequency and intensity of the disorder, the settings in which the disorder occurs, who interacted with the child, and the conditions before and after an episode, especially social interactions that are potential reinforcers. A recording chart such as the one shown in Figure 1.3 should be provided to parents or health care personnel who are responsible for the child during baseline assessment. This chart should also be used during all treatment phases. In addition, a graph showing the frequency of episodes per day or week should be kept in the child's home or hospital setting as a record of treatment progress.

After a week of baseline data collection, the parents and therapist should be able to see that some conditions systematically occur before or after the child's disorder episodes. These may be contributing to the intensity and frequency of behavior or apparent symptoms, according to behavioral prin-

FIGURE 1.3. Recording chart for baseline and treatment recording

BEHAVIORAL/MEDICAL RECORDING CHART

Name _____ Date _____ Disorder: Behavioral

Problem _____

Duration of   Medical

Time _____ Episode _____ Problem _____

ANTECEDENT CONDITIONS

Child's Behavior _____

Parent's Behavior _____

Other's Behavior _____

Medical Intervention _____

Behavioral Intervention _____

EPISODE

Behavior Intensity-Low Med Hi   Comments: _____

Apparent Symptom Intensity-Low Med Hi   _____

Setting _____

CONSEQUENCES

Parent Reaction _____

Other Reaction _____

Behavioral Intervention _____

Medical Treatment _____

Child's Behavior _____

Child's Emotion _____

ciples as applied to the systems shown in Figure 1.1. A tentative behavioral and medical diagnosis of the disorder can now be made, which should have direct implications for treatment. The diagnosis is tentative since it can only be confirmed through successful application of the behavioral techniques. Ultimate success may require reintervention since the baseline assessment and hypotheses of behavioral control derived from it could be in error.

As shown in Figure 1.2, the medical and behavioral aspects of the disorder may be assessed independently, but the medical and behavioral treatments must be developed in a collaborative fashion, since they may have an interactive effect on the child. For example, sleep onset insomnia may have an operant component in that the child's presleep behaviors are reinforced through parental attention. If normal doses of narcoleptic drugs are part of the therapy plan, sleep may occur promptly. However, this eliminates the possibility of modifying the child-parent reinforcement system, since the target behavior no longer occurs while drug therapy is effective. The behavioral treatment might involve having the parents extinguish inappropriate presleep behaviors by systematically ignoring them. If the child's behaviors increase in intensity as an initial response to extinction, the narcoleptic drugs could be prescribed for the parents, to help them ignore the child. A mild sedative may mitigate the child's reactions and at the same time provide the conditions necessary for extinction to occur. From this example, it can be seen that a careful titration of the effects of medical and behavioral treatment is necessary. Especially in disorders involving pain, asthma, seizures, sleep, or hyperactivity, such titration is needed. A purely medical approach may have limitations, including side effects, drug tolerance, and attribution effects; a purely behavioral approach may mask undetected physiological problems. The optimal solution in terms of the comfort and health of the child may involve some palliative medication even if the behavioral treatment by itself produces appropriate behavior. The amount of negative affect expressed by the child would be a criterion for assessing appropriate treatment. Each case of this type should be considered as a multiple-baseline case study (Hersen & Barlow, 1976). Behavioral effects can be separated from medical effects by applying the techniques sequentially and allowing for stabilization of behaviors and symptoms before another change is made in either treatment modality. In Figure 1.2 the "short-term evaluation" is the point where this titration occurs. After several iterations of successive modifications of medical and behavioral treatments, a final treatment package can be prescribed for long-term implementation. The short-term evaluation should include some measure of compliance to treatment recommendations. Since parental reports may be biased or inaccurate, objective observers in the natural settings might be employed with particularly difficult disorders, especially if family disturbance is suspected. After compliance has been assessed, treatment effects can be evaluated. While medication may produce various side effects, behavioral treatments may result in symptom substitution. For example, if the target behaviors or symptoms are reinforced by attention, an extinction paradigm may provoke other behaviors or symptoms as the child strives for attention through other methods. If the behavioral techniques are applied to these new behaviors, the child should learn that his new attempts will be ineffective.

Once the medical and behavioral techniques have been tried out and have been found to be effective in the primary treatment setting (hospital or home), then these same or slightly modified techniques should be applied in the other settings in which the child normally lives. This generalization procedure is especially necessary for younger or developmentally retarded children for whom the primary treatment setting may provide discriminative stimuli that are not present in other settings. Older, more developed children who understand the purpose of their treatment can more easily generalize their improvements across settings. Setting variables include different social situations as well as different physical locations; a father or teacher may not be able to elicit appropriate behavior from a child who is already under control of the mother. An excellent review of generalization research and theory can be found in the work of Wahler, Berland, and Coe (1979).

Given that appropriate behavior and a satisfactory physical condition are attained across the child's various settings, it must then be assured that the modifications are maintained indefinitely. Some of the factors that may affect maintenance of appropriate behaviors on the part of all persons involved in therapy (including child, parent, pediatrician, and behavior therapist) include:

1. Perceived self-efficacy of persons involved to achieve treatment goals
2. Degree of perceived success toward goals after an initial treatment period
3. Perceived difficulty and expense of techniques
4. Perceived usefulness of techniques
5. Unrealistic expectations
6. Preparedness in case of temporary relapse (Foreyt and Goodrick, in press)

Thus it is clear that the parent and child should feel that the treatment techniques will work and that they are able to perform them. They need to understand the limitations of the techniques, and know what to do in case of reversion to former ways of behaving. These cognitive conditions can be assessed through interviews before the therapist and pediatrician allow the child and his family to enter into a period of self-management without regular clinical help.

Marholin and Siegel (1978) have outlined strategies to ensure maintenance of behavior change. According to them, the behavioral control techniques used during the maintenance period should be similar to those used to obtain the initial behavior change. All persons who interact with the child should be familiar with the techniques. Social reinforcers should replace material reinforcers soon so that appropriate behaviors can come under control of naturally occurring social responses. If considerable reinforcement is needed initially, it should be gradually decreased to the rate found in a normal setting, and the delay between performance and reward should gradually approximate what the child can expect in a normal life. Children who are mature enough can be taught to control the antecedents and consequences of their own behavior, and to internalize judgments of their performances so that they self-control appropriate behavior. Finally, Marholin and Siegel suggest that children should be made to feel that their successes and failures are the result of their own actions. This should allow self-correcting cognitions to develop.

Finally, the last step shown in Figure 1.2 is the long-term follow-up. Many behavioral approaches have demonstrated short-term change while ignoring long-term maintenance of behavior change (Keeley, Shemberg, & Carbonell, 1976). Long-term compliance with the medical regimen is also a problem (Becker & Maiman, 1975). No treatment can be deemed a success unless it has lasting effects; in many pediatric behavioral medicine treatments, tracking the progress of the child for a year or even more may be required to substantiate the efficacy of the treatment. Furthermore, the evaluation of treatment should go beyond the specific disorder corrected. Changes in social and academic functioning as well as affect and personality characteristics are all potentially changed by the correction of a partially disabling behavioral or medical problem. According to the systems model presented in Figure 1.1, evaluation of family therapy may also be needed.

Such evaluation procedures are important for at least two reasons. First, many of the areas covered in this volume lack vigorous experimental tests for the behavioral treatments used; most of the reports are case studies. Special features of case studies may make easy generalization to other cases problematic. Second, many of the studies in this field were done in university research settings, with many of the children's families self-selected from higher socioeconomic strata. The expectations for success of highly funded and exhaustively detailed research may have been very high, especially as these techniques are considered innovative. These high expectations, together with the greater ability of highly educated parents to carry out the treatment recommendations, may have resulted in a higher success rate than would be the case for normal pediatric behavioral medicine as applied to lower socioeconomic families whose parenting skills and social circumstances do not allow for optimal treatment conditions. Indeed McAuley and McAuley (1977) report that the overall success rate for behavioral treatment of children may be below 50 percent.

In summary, when a health professional deals with a problem in pediatric behavioral medicine, all the steps shown in Figure 1.2 should be undertaken with care. At each step a behavioral systems analysis should be done following the systems model shown in Figure 1.1. For the proper growth of the field of pediatric behavioral medicine, detailed records should be kept for each step, and multiple case studies using demonstrated effective procedures should be published. It is to be hoped that health care facilities will increasingly integrate medical and behavioral resources so that all aspects of childhood disorders can be properly treated.

FUTURE STATUS OF PEDIATRIC BEHAVIORAL MEDICINE

An impressive number of research studies have demonstrated the efficacy of many of these behavioral techniques in the treatment of childhood problems. Unlike many other therapists, behavior therapists, as an integral part of their technology, regularly collect and use objective data to formulate and modify their therapeutic interventions. This collection of data exposes them to the failures and successes of their treatment regimen. Though behavior therapists may at times be resistant to following the direction of their data, they have been most active in incisively identifying the problems and failures of their techniques. In general, behavior therapists have been their own worst critics and have used their feedback systems to direct new research efforts toward more effective treatment techniques.

Behavior therapists are becoming increasingly aware of the complexity of human behavior and the interactive characteristics of therapeutic interventions as indicated in the systems model. They are increasing work with children in the natural environment, enlisting members of the nuclear and extended family in the treatment process, and attempting to provide preventive educational experiences for the major societal change agents— parents, teachers, pediatricians, pastors, parole officers, and so on. Behavior therapists no longer believe that the manipulation of a few simple variables will permanently alter behavior. They have learned that complex human behavior demands complex strategies and have effectively utilized their data to direct how these strategies will be applied. They have learned that reinforcers vary from setting to setting and are influenced by such non-behavioral, internal processes as expectancy.

In the future, behavior therapists will continue to extend their analysis, research, and treatment techniques not only out into the natural environment but also internally, relating autonomic, neurological, and physiological processes to the behavior change process. In the present state of development of our behavioral technology, we are at a primarily descriptive and analytic phase and are faced with the complexity and specificity of human behavior in its multidetermined and interactive nature. Out of this descriptive phase should emerge some summary principles of an effective behavior change technology.

REFERENCES

Adelson, R., & Goldfried, M. R. Modeling and the fearful child patient. *Journal of Dentistry for Children*, 1970, *37*, 34-37.

Alexander, A. D., Chai, H., Creer, T. L., Miklich, D. R., Renee, C. M., & de A. Cardosa, R. The elimination of chronic cough by response suppression shaping. *Journal of Behavior Therapy and Experimental Psychiatry*, 1973, *4*, 75-80.

Alford, G. S., Blanchard, E. B., & Buckley, T. M. Treatment of hysterical vomiting by modification of social contingencies: A case study. *Journal of Behavior Therapy and Experimental Psychiatry*, 1972, *3*, 209-212.

Allen, K. E., & Harris, F. R. Elimination of a child's excessive scratching by training the mother in reinforcement procedures. *Behaviour Research and Therapy*, 1966, *4*, 79-84.

Atkeson, B. M., & Forehand, R. Parent behavioral training for problem children: An examination of studies using multiple outcome measures. *Journal of Abnormal Child Psychology*, 1978, *6*, 449-460.

Ayllon, T., Layman, D., & Kandel, H. J. A behavioral-educational alternative to drug control of hyperactive children. *Journal of Applied Behavior Analysis*, 1975, *8*, 137-146.

Azrin, N. H., & Nunn, R. G. Habit-reversal: A method of eliminating nervous habits and tics. *Behaviour Research and Therapy*, 1973, *11*, 619-628.

Azrin, N. H., & Nunn, R. G. A rapid method of eliminating stuttering by a regulated breathing approach. *Behaviour Research and Therapy*, 1974, *12*, 279-286.

Azrin, N. H., Sneed, T. J., & Foxx, R. M. Dry-bed training: Rapid elimination of childhood enuresis. *Behaviour Research and Therapy*, 1974, *12*, 147-156.

Baer, D. M. Laboratory control of thumb sucking by withdrawal and representation of reinforcement. *Journal of the Experimental Analysis of Behavior*, 1962, *5*, 525-528.

Baer, D. M. Remedial use of the reinforcement contingency. Paper presented at the Annual Convention of the American Psychological Association, Chicago, 1966.

Bandura, A. *Principles of behavior modification.* New York: Holt, Rinehart & Winston, 1969.

Bandura, A. *Social learning theory.* Englewood Cliffs, N.J.: Prentice Hall, 1976.

Bär, L. H. J., & Kuypers, B. R. M. Behaviour therapy in dermatological practice. *British Journal of Dermatology*, 1973, *88*, 591-598.

Bates, J. E., Skilbeck, W. M., Smith, K. V. R., & Bentler, P. M. Intervention with families of gender-disturbed boys. *American Journal of Orthopsychiatry*, 1975, *45*, 150-157.

Becker, M. H., & Maiman, L. A. Sociobehavioral determinants of compliance with health and medical care recommendations. *Medical Care*, 1975, *13*, 10-24.

Becker, W. C. *Parents are teachers: A child management program.* Champaign, Ill.: Research Press, 1971.

Becker, W. C. Application of behavioral principles in typical classrooms. In The National Society for the Study of Education (Ed.), *Seventy-second Yearbook of the National Society for the Study of Education.* Chicago: University of Chicago Press, 1973.

Bentler, P. M. A note on the treatment of adolescent sex problems. *Journal of Child Psychology and Psychiatry,* 1968, *9,* 125-129.

Berkowitz, B. P., & Graziano, A. M. Training parents as behavior therapists: A review. *Behaviour Research and Therapy,* 1972, *10,* 297-317.

Bernal, M. E. Behavioral feedback in the modification of brat behaviors. *Journal of Nervous and Mental Disease,* 1969, *148,* 375-385.

Buckley, N. K., & Walker, H. M. *Modifying classroom behavior: A manual of procedures for classroom teachers.* Champaign, Ill.: Research Press, 1970.

Clement, P. W. Please, mother, I'd rather you did it yourself: Training parents to treat their own children. Paper presented at the meeting of the Western Psychological Association, Los Angeles, California, 1970.

DeLeon, G., & Mandell, W. A comparison of conditioning and psychotherapy in the treatment of functional enuresis. *Journal of Clinical Psychology,* 1966, *22,* 326-330.

Drash, P. W. Behavior modification: New tools for use in pediatric dentistry with the handicapped child. *Dental Clinics of North America,* 1971, *18,* 617-631.

Foreyt, J. P., & Goodrick, G. K. Assessment of childhood obesity. In E. Mash & L. Terdal (Eds.), *Behavior assessment of childhood disorders.* New York: Guilford Press, in press.

Garber, N. B. Operant procedures to eliminate drooling behavior in a cerebral palsied adolescent. *Developmental Medicine and Child Neurology,* 1971, *13,* 641-644.

Gardner, J. E. Behavioral therapy treatment approach to a psychogenic seizure disorder. *Journal of Consulting Psychology,* 1967, *31,* 209-212.

Garrard, K. R., & Saxon, S. A. Preparation of a disturbed deaf child for therapy: A case description in behavior shaping. *Journal of Speech and Hearing Disorders,* 1973, *38,* 502-509.

Graziano, A. M. *Programmed therapy: The development of group behavioral approaches to severely disturbed children.* New York: Pergamon, 1971.

Graziano, A. M. Parents as behavior therapist. In M. Hersen, R. M. Eisler, & P. M. Miller (Eds.), *Progress in behavior modification* (Vol. 5). New York: Academic Press, 1977.

Hall, R. V. *Managing behavior: Part I. The measurement of behavior.* Lawrence, Kansas: H and H Enterprises, 1971.

Hall, R. V., Axelrod, S., Tyler, L., Grief, E., Jones, F. C., & Robertson, R. Modification of behavior problems in the home with a parent as observer and experimenter. *Journal of Applied Behavior Analysis,* 1972, *5,* 53-64.

Hanf, C. A two-stage program for modifying maternal controlling during mother-child (M-C) interaction. Paper presented at the meeting of the Western Psychological Association, Vancouver, B.C., 1969.

Hart, B. M., Reynolds, N. J., Baer, D. M., Brawley, E. R., & Harris, F. R. Effect of contingent and non-contingent social reinforcement on the cooperative play of a preschool child. *Journal of Applied Behavior Analysis*, 1968, *1*, 73-76.

Hersen, M., & Barlow, D. H. *Single-case experimental designs: Strategies for studying behavior change*. New York: Pergamon Press, 1976.

Hewett, F. M. *The emotionally disturbed child in the classroom: A developmental strategy for educating children with maladaptive behavior*. Boston: Allyn and Bacon, 1969.

Homme, L., Csanyi, A. P., Gonzales, M. A., & Rechs, J. R. *How to use contingency contracting in the classroom*. Champaign, Ill.: Research Press, 1969.

Homme, L., & Tosti, D. *Behavior technology: Motivation and contingency management*. San Rafael, California: Individual Learning System, 1971.

Hutzell, R. R., Platzek, D., & Logue, P. E. Control of symptoms of Gilles de la Tourette's syndrome by self-monitoring. *Journal of Behavior Therapy and Experimental Psychiatry*, 1974, *5*, 71-76.

Ince, L. P. The use of relaxation training and a conditioned stimulus in the elimination of epileptic seizures in a child: A case study. *Journal of Behavior Therapy and Experimental Psychiatry*, 1976, *7*, 39-42.

Johnson, C. A., & Katz, R. C. Using parents as change agents for their children: A review. *Journal of Child Psychology and Psychiatry*, 1973, *14*, 181-200.

Keeley, S. M., Shemberg, K. M., & Carbonell, J. Operant clinical intervention: Behavior management or beyond? Where are the data? *Behavior Therapy*, 1976, *7*, 292-305.

Kennedy, W. A. School phobia: Rapid treatment of fifty cases. *Journal of Abnormal Psychology*, 1965, *70*, 285-289.

Lal, J., & Lindsley, O. R. Therapy of chronic constipation in a young child by rearranging social contingencies. *Behaviour Research and Therapy* 1968, *6*, 484-485.

Liebman, R., Minuchin, S., & Baker, L. The use of structured family therapy in the treatment of tractable asthma. *American Journal of Psychiatry*, 1974, *131*, 535-540.

Lovibond, S. H. *Conditioning and enuresis*. Oxford: Pergamon, 1964.

Madsen, C. H., Jr., Becker, W. C., Thomas, D. R., Kosar, L., & Plager, E. An analysis of the reinforcing function of "sit down" commands. In R. K. Parker (Ed.), *Readings in educational psychology*. Boston: Allyn and Bacon, 1968.

Madsen, C. H., Jr., & Madsen, C. K. *Teaching-discipline: A positive approach for educational development* (2nd ed.). Boston: Allyn and Bacon, 1975.

Mahoney, M. J. *Cognition and behavior modification*. Cambridge, Mass.: Ballinger, 1974.

Marholin, D., & Siegel, L. T. Beyond the law of effect: Programming for the maintenance of behavioral change. In D. Marholin (Ed.), *Child behavior therapy*. New York: Gardner Press, 1978.

McAuley, R., & McAuley, P. *Child behavior problems: An empirical approach to management.* New York: The Free Press, 1977.

McLaughlin, J. G., & Nay, W. R. Treatment of trichotillomania using positive coverants and response cost: A case report. *Behavior Therapy,* 1975, *6,* 87-91.

Meichenbaum, D. H. *Cognitive behavior modification.* New York: Plenum, 1977.

Meichenbaum, D. H., & Goodman, J. Teaching impulsive children to talk to themselves: A means of developing self control. *Journal of Abnormal Psychology,* 1971, *77,* 115-126.

Miller, A. J., & Kratochwill, T. R. Reduction of frequent stomachache complaints by time out. *Behavior Therapy,* 1979, *10,* 211-218.

Miller, A. L. Treatment of a child with Gilles de la Tourette's syndrome using behavior modification techniques. *Journal of Behavior Therapy and Experimental Psychiatry.* 1970, *1,* 319-321.

Mira, M. Behavioral modification applied to training young deaf children. *Exceptional Children,* 1972, *10,* 225-229.

Neisworth, J. T., Madle, R. A., & Goeke, K. E. "Errorless" elimination of separation anxiety: A case study. *Journal of Behavior Therapy and Experimental Psychiatry,* 1975, *6,* 79-82.

Neisworth, J. T., & Moore, F. Operant treatment of asthmatic responding with the parent as therapist. *Behavior Therapy,* 1972, *3,* 95-99.

O'Dell, S. Training parents in behavior modification: A review. *Psychological Bulletin,* 1974, *81,* 418-433.

O'Leary, K. D., O'Leary, S., & Becker, W. C. Modification of a deviant sibling interaction pattern in the home. *Behaviour Research and Therapy,* 1967. *5,* 113-120.

Ollendick, T. H., & Gruen, C. E. Treatment of a bodily injury phobia with implosive therapy. *Journal of Consulting and Clinical Psychology,* 1972, *38,* 389-393.

Palmer, S., Thompson, R. J., & Linscheid, T. R. Applied behavior analysis in the treatment of childhood feeding problems. *Developmental Medicine and Child Neurology,* 1975, *17,* 333-339.

Patterson, G. R. *Families.* Champaign, Ill.: Research Press, 1971a.

Patterson, G. R. Behavioral intervention procedures in the classroom and in the home. In A. E. Bergin & S. L. Garfield (Eds.), *Handbook of Psychotherapy and behavior change: An empirical analysis.* New York: Wiley, 1971b.

Patterson, G. R. Interventions for boys with conduct problems: Multiple settings, treatments and criteria. *Journal of Consulting and Clinical Psychology,* 1974, *42,* 471-481.

Patterson, G. R., Cobb, J. A., & Ray, R. A. A social engineering technology for retraining the families of aggressive boys. In H. E. Adams & I. P. Unikel (Eds.), *Issues and trends in behavior therapy.* Springfield, Ill.: Charles D. Thomas, 1973.

Patterson, G. R., & Gullion, M. E. *Living with children* (Rev.ed.). Champaign, Ill.: Research Press, 1971.

Rekers, G. A., Lovaas, O. I., & Low, B. The behavioral treatment of a "transsexual" preadolescent boy. *Journal of Abnormal Child Psychology*, 1974, *2*, 99-116.

Renne, C. M., & Creer, T. L. Training children with asthma to use inhalation therapy equipment. *Journal of Applied Behavioral Analysis*, 1976, *9*, 1-11.

Rosen, M., & Wesner, C. Case report: A behavioral approach to Tourette's syndrome. *Journal of Consulting and Clinical Psychology*, 1973, *41*, 308-312.

Ross, D. M., Ross, S. A., & Evans, T. A. The modification of extreme social withdrawal by modeling with guided participation. *Journal of Behavior Therapy and Experimental Psychiatry*, 1971, *2*, 273-279.

Sajwaj, T., Libet, J., & Agras, S. Lemon-juice therapy: A control of life-threatening rumination in a six-month-old infant. *Journal of Applied Behavior Analysis*, 1974, *7*, 557-563.

Sanok, R. L. & Streifel, S. Elective mutism: Generalization of verbal responding across people and settings. *Behavior Therapy*, 1979, *10*, 357-371.

Schroeder, C. S. Psychologist in a private pediatric practice. *Journal of Pediatric Psychology*, 1979, *4*, 5-18.

Schwartz, G. E., & Weiss, S. M. Yale conference on behavioral medicine: A proposed definition and statement of goals. *Journal of Behavioral Medicine*, 1978, *1*, 3-12.

Shorkey, C. T., & Taylor, J. E. Management of maladaptive behavior of a severely burned child. *Child Welfare*, 1973, *52*, 543-547.

Stark, J., Rosenbaum, R. L., Schwartz, D., & Wisan, A. The non-verbal child: Some clinical guidelines. *Journal of Speech and Hearing Disorders*, 1973, *38*, 59-71.

Stuart, R. B. Behavioral contracting within the family of delinquents. *Journal of Behavior Therapy and Experimental Psychiatry*, 1971, *2*, 1-11.

Toepfer, C., Reuter, J., & Maurer, C. Design and evaluation of an obedience training program for mothers of pre-school children. *Journal of Consulting and Clinical Psychology*, 1972, *39*, 194-198.

Ulan, H., Juris, A., & Dornback, F. Keeping that patch on: The application of behavior modification techniques in orthoptic practice. *American Orthoptic Journal*, 1974, *34*, 60-62.

Wagner, M. K. A case of public masturbation treated by operant conditioning. *Journal of Child Psychology and Psychiatry*, 1968, *9*, 61-65.

Wahler, R. G., Berland, R. M., & Coe, T. D. Generalization processes in child behavior change. In B. B. Lahey & A. E. Kazdin (Eds.), *Advances in clinical child psychology* (Vol. 2). New York: Plenum, 1979.

Wahler, R. G., Winkel, G. H., Peterson, R. F., & Morrison, D. C. Mothers as behavior therapists for their own children. *Behaviour Research and Therapy*, 1965, *3*, 113-124.

Walder, L. O., Cohen, S. I., Breiter, D. E., Warman, F. C., Orme-Johnson, D., & Pavey, S. Parents as agents of behavior change. In S. E. Golann & C. Eisdorfer (Eds.), *Handbook of community mental health*. New York: Appleton-Century-Crofts, 1972.

Weil, G., & Goldfried, M. R.   Treatment of insomnia in an eleven-year-old child through self-relaxation. *Behavior Therapy*, 1973, *4*, 282-294.

Wheeler, M. E., & Hess, K. W.   Treatment of juvenile obesity by successive approximation control of eating. *Journal of Behavior Therapy and Experimental Psychiatry*, 1976, *7*, 235-241.

Wolf, M., Risley, T., & Mees, H.   Application of operant conditioning procedures to the behavior problems of an autistic child. *Behaviour Therapy and Research*, 1964, *1*, 305-312.

Wright, L., Woodcock, J., & Scott, R.   Treatment of sleep disturbance in a young child by conditioning. *Southern Medical Journal*, 1970, *63*, 174-176.

Zeilberger, J., Sampen, S. E., & Sloane, H. N., Jr.   Modification of a child's problem behaviors in the home with the mother as therapist. *Journal of Applied Behavior Analysis.* 1968, *1*, 47-53.

Zifferblatt, S. M.   *Improving study and homework behaviors.* Champaign, Ill.: Research Press, 1970.

Zlutnick, S., Mayville, W. J., & Moffat, S.   Modification of seizure disorders: The interruption of behavioral chains. *Journal of Applied Behavior Analysis*, 1975, *8*, 1-12.

2

DERMATOLOGY

INTRODUCTION

Skin

Disorders of the skin and emotional states are generally recognized as interrelated. Stress frequently causes or aggravates inflammatory skin conditions. In addition to prescribing topical medications, systemic drugs, sedatives, and tranquilizers, physicians frequently resort to instructions to "rub, not scratch" and, if a condition is severe enough they may apply casts or special splints. Traditional, psychodynamic therapies are a useful adjunct to the long-term management of dermatological disorders, but offer little for the immediate management of skin problems. Children who suffer skin disorders must cope with the embarrassing evidence of their disorder, and with the continuous stress of itching, medication, and frequent reminders to stop scratching. These take their toll in immediate personal comfort and long-term self-enhancement.

In their section of the chapter, Bär and Kuypers (1973) describe the application of behavior therapies to a wide variety of dermatological disorders. Neurodermatitis, lichen simplex, trichotillomania, chronic eczema, blushing, and severe palmer hyperhidrosis (sweating) were treated by a combination of relaxation training, systematic desensitization, social skills and assertive training, token economies, and contingent use of attention.

Atopic dermatitis accounts for 20 percent of patients treated for dermatological disorders. Atopic children frequently have "sensitive skin" and a family history of asthma, hay fever, migraine headaches, or hyperactivity. Some of these children respond to normal environmental stimulation with excessive irritation and dry skin; others, under stress at home or school, begin to scratch dry skin created by excessive autonomic activation. The net result is the beginning of an "itch-scratch-itch" cycle. Once the scratching begins, regardless of its specific etiology, it becomes quite resistant to extinction. The pleasurable aspects of itching as well as attention from parents and physician provide reinforcement for this undesired behavior. Attempts to exercise self-control to create extinction of the scratching response generally lead to a worsening of the skin condition. Without support of a therapeutic relationship, the child's nonscratching behavior seldom persists long enough to allow extinction and healing to occur.

Allen and Harris (1966), in their classic article, describe the session-by-session treatment of a five-year-old child's excessive scratching. Therapy consisted of training the parents, mainly the mother, in the use of positive reinforcement techniques. This article not only illustrates the importance of a thorough behavioral analysis and careful monitoring, but also emphasizes the importance of behavioral treatment occurring within the context of a supportive relationship.

Burns

Children with extensive burns represent significant management difficulties for physicians and allied health personnel. Nover (1973) regards the burned child's reaction to pain as the most significant factor contributing to difficult hospital management. Bernstein (1965) suggests the use of hypnosis as a way of decreasing anxiety. Labaw (1973) describes the use of hypnosis, along with relaxation training and game playing to reduce anxiety and induce cooperation.

Zide and Pardoe (1976) present a case study of a 13-year-old child with second- and third-degree burns. Because of the adolescent's generally uncooperative and manipulative behaviors, the management of the child was placed in the hands of one physician and a reward system was instituted for adherence to the ward routine and to the treatment regimen. After five weeks of treatment, the patient was able to sleep without medication and was recovering acceptably.

Woodward and Jackson (1961) have stressed the importance of communication not only between physician and patient but also between physician and parents. Young, verbal children must understand the treatment procedures and the extent of their required cooperation. Preverbal children who are treated for burns must have some means of discriminating between feeding and caring functions and the painful treatment functions. Woodward and Jackson suggest that both parents and children be helped to understand how the burns occurred. Any misinterpretation on the part of the children may lead to hostile and aggressive feelings either toward themselves or toward their parents.

In this section Shorkey and Taylor (1973) recount the management strategies, primarily discrimination training, for a 17-month-old child with second- and third-degree burns over 37 percent of her body. After four months of treatment, the child's physical condition had deteriorated because of her refusal to eat. Skin grafts were ineffective due to her excessive crying and motility. Motor agitation began when the staff approached either for therapeutic reasons or for pleasurable activities. Behavioral observation revealed the child's inability to discriminate between personnel providing painful treatment procedures and those involved in care and feeding. A discrimination procedure was set up, with treatment personnel wearing green isolation gowns, quickly and efficiently performing their treatment without interacting with the child, and other personnel wearing red, sterilized bags at times of feeding, body massage, and other play activities. After two weeks the child was responding to treatment, smiling, and playing games. She was discharged after six weeks.

The use of both operant and respondent behavioral techniques have outstanding potential as primary and secondary treatment modalities in dealing with common dermatological problems. As one component of a multifaceted medical procedure, these strategies can be used to increase adherence to treatment, decrease cost and length of hospitalization, and minimize the development of maladaptive behavioral patterns that might persist after the medical problem is treated.

References

Allen, K. E., & Harris, F. R. Elimination of a child's excessive scratching by training the mother in reinforcement procedures. *Behaviour Research and Therapy*, 1966, *4*, 79-84.

Bär, L. H. J., & Kuypers, B. R. M. Behaviour therapy in dermatological practice. *British Journal of Dermatology*, 1973, *88*, 591-598.

Bernstein, N. R. Observations on the use of hypnosis with burned children on a pediatric ward. *International Journal of Clinical Experimental Hypnosis*, 1965, *13*, 1-10.

Labaw, W. L. Adjunctive trance therapy with severely burned children. *International Journal of Child Psychotherapy*, 1973, *2*, 80-92.

Nover, R. A. Pain and the burned child. *Journal of Academy of Child Psychiatry*, 1973, *12*, 499-505.

Shorkey, C. T., & Taylor, J. E. Management of maladaptive behavior of a severely burned child. *Child Welfare*, 1973, *52*, 543-547.

Woodward, J., & Jackson, D. Emotional reactions in burnt children and their mothers. *British Journal of Plastic Surgery*, 1961, *13*, 316-324.

Zide, B., & Pardoe, R. The use of behavioral modification therapy in a recalcitrant burned child. *Plastic and Reconstructive Surgery*, 1976, *57*, 378-382.

BEHAVIOUR THERAPY
IN DERMATOLOGICAL PRACTICE

Louis H. J. Bär
Ben R. M. Kuypers

SUMMARY

Behaviour therapy provides important psychotherapeutic possibilities for the treatment of dermatological disorders. Compulsive scratching and trichotillomania can be treated by aversive conditioning, or by the token economy technique. The treatment of blushing is described: assertive training is useful for patients with symptomatic erythema and erythrophobia. Hyperhidrosis can be treated by assertive training and systematic desensitization.

A new and important addition to the therapeutic possibilities available to the psychotherapist treating dermatological patients is the recently developed technique of *behaviour therapy*. Behaviour, or conditioning, therapy uses experimentally established principles of learning for the purpose of changing unadaptive behaviour. This unadaptive or neurotic behaviour is seen as a consequence of a faulty learning process and the aim of treatment is to weaken or eliminate them and to initiate and strengthen adaptive habits (Wolpe, 1969).

METHODS

The various techniques of behaviour therapy used in dermatological practice may be grouped into four main divisions.

Reprinted from the *British Journal of Dermatology*, 1973, *88*, 591-598. Reprinted by permission.

Louis H. J. Bär is at the Institute for Medical Psychotherapy, Utrecht, Holland. Ben R. M. Kuypers is at Biseweide 34, Grubbemvorst, Holland.

Systematic desensitization

This is used mainly in neurotic disorders in which anxiety is a prominent feature. This method is described by Wolpe (1969): "It is the breaking down of neurotic anxiety-response habits in piecemeal fashion. A psychological state inhibitory of anxiety is induced in the patient, who is then exposed to a weak anxiety-arousing stimulus. The exposure is repeated until the stimulus loses completely its ability to evoke anxiety. Then progressively 'stronger' stimuli are introduced and similarly treated. This technique, which characteristically employs relaxation on the anxiety-inhibiting state, has made it possible for the first time to exert direct control over a great many neurotic habits."

Aversion therapy

This is used in the treatment of persistent behaviour disorders, such as compulsive scratching. The method consists of giving an electric shock whenever the unadaptive habit is demonstrated or displayed.

Operant techniques

These are also used to modify compulsive habits. Adaptive behaviour is reinforced by giving a reward; unadaptive behaviour is weakened or eliminated by being neglected or even punished.

Assertive training

This is used in patients who dare not express their emotions and who experience extreme or considerable social fear. The training consists in teaching them to behave more frankly towards the rising fear, and in that way to overcome it.

A full description of these methods and their theoretical backgrounds has been given by Wolpe (1969), Bandura (1969), Yates (1970) and Lazarus (1971).

CASE REPORTS

Compulsive Scratching

Psychological investigation of patients with neurodermatitis sometimes reveals conflict situations or emotional problems. According to psychoanalytically or other psychodynamically oriented theories these conflicts have been alleged to be the *cause* of scratching. Behaviour therapy, however, approaches these problems from another viewpoint. Walton (1960), for instance, concludes after examining a woman with neurodermatitis and compulsive scratching "that the skin condition may well have originated because of physical considerations, though its *continuance* might have been perpetuated by psychological factors, the understanding and treatment of which could be formulated in terms of learning theory. The rewards initially associated with the continuance of the neurodermatitis had reinforced scratching until it had become a powerful compulsive habit and it was this which had therefore directly perpetuated the skin condition." The attention that the patient got from her environment, because of her scratching, was the reinforcement which maintained the scratching. *Ignoring* this unwanted behaviour resulted in a decrease of the scratching until it stopped altogether. This reduction corresponded with a gradual improvement in the neurodermatitis which disappeared at the end of 3 months and did not return within 4 years. In conditioning terms, stopping the reinforcement of the neurotic behaviour resulted in extinction of the undesired and unadaptive habit.

It is also possible, though, to *reward* the desired behaviour (non-scratching). This form of *operant conditioning* also appears to be very useful in the treatment of compulsive behaviour and may be used in combination with ignoring the existing behaviour. In principle the method consists of rewarding the patient for not having scratched for a certain period of time. Because it is in practice very difficult to give a valid reward every time, one can use secondary reinforcers or tokens. With this method, the *token economy* system, the patient receives a token after a short fixed interval, for instance an hour (dependent on the schedule or reinforcement). If after a longer period he has still not scratched, for instance a day, he may hand in a fixed number of tokens (secondary reinforcement) in return for a very attractive reward (primary reinforcement). With the help of this method compulsive scratching, especially in *children*, can be unlearned within a relatively short time.

Allen & Harris (1966) described the treatment by such a method of a girl aged 5 with excessive scratching. These authors are of the opinion, after a 3 year study, that "problem behaviour of normal children was controlled by its immediate consequence, the attention of adults." It is important then "to teach parents to modify their own attending behaviour in ways that might then resolve their child's problem." The authors persuaded the parents to ignore scratching and to reinforce desirable behaviour (non-scratching) by tokens. They report that at the end of 6 weeks the child's face and body were clear of all scabs and sores. As the scratching decreased, the mother was instructed in appropriate techniques for reducing the reinforcement schedule. Four months later the scratching behaviour had not recurred. Our treatment procedure and results correspond with those described by Allen & Harris.

Case 1. A girl aged 6 with severe neurodermatitis of the vulva had scratched herself day and night for 3 years. After the disappearance of the physical cause (Oxyuris), the scratching persisted. Two periods in hospital had no success. The girl was a hyperactive, restless child who demanded much attention from the environment. The mother was a rather rationalistic woman, who frequently discussed the scratching with the patient and who had tried many remedies for this behaviour. We hypothesized that the scratching behaviour was a form of attention seeking by the child, in which this unadaptive behaviour was at the same time reinforced by the attention received by it from the environment. The treatment plan involved giving the child the necessary positive attention, not as a result of scratching, but rather as a reward for not scratching. The mother was given instructions to ignore completely all scratching behaviour and to give attention to the child at the moments of non-scratching. Each hour the child received a token if scratching had been absent during that period. During schooltime the programme was continued in the same way. Every evening the girl could exchange the tokens of the day for a sweet. For the night period she always had a favourite and valued toy to look forward to. After 5 weeks she scratched distinctly less during the night and after 13 weeks the programme could be stopped (Figure 2.1). 18 months' follow-up showed no relapses. In conditioning terms, stopping the reinforcement of the neurotic behaviour and reinforcing the desired behaviour resulted in extinction of the undesired and unadaptive habit.

Sometimes the psychologist can find no psychological or social problems which maintain the compulsive behaviour, yet the patient scratches and often the neurodermatitis spreads further. A close analysis will then often show that, here too, the scratching has had a physical cause, which has now disappeared, whereas the scratching persists. The positive reinforcement which perpetuates the scratching appears thus to be the abolition of the unbearable itch (tension) and in consequence tension reduction. By scratching, the itch diminishes, which is an enjoyable experience, which again reinforces the urge to scratch. In this way a vicious circle is set up. In such a case it is reasonable to break the vicious circle by stopping the act of scratching from being enjoyable, that is to make it unpleasant, and thus to evoke in the patient an aversion against scratching.

Such a method is described by Ratliff & Stein (1968). They treated a patient with severe neurodermatitis. The treatment plan involved *aversive conditioning* procedures. The authors gave the subject an electric shock (I mA) whenever he scratched any part of his body. The shock was terminated immediately after he stopped scratching and said aloud, "Don't scratch." An alternative, but complementary, treatment approach was adopted by the authors in the hope of establishing more permanent and general therapeutic effects. This approach involved training the patient in progressive relaxation with instructions to apply this technique each time he experienced the "urge to scratch." It was hypothesized that relaxation should serve to compete with the unpleasant sensations resulting from not scratching, and either to maintain or facilitate the acquisition of alternative responses incompatible with scratching. After about 5 weeks under this treatment the maladaptive scratching had been completely eliminated and did not return within the 6 months follow-up. Our own method of aversion therapy is a variation of this.

Case 2. A man aged 33 suffered from severe lichen simplex on the scrotum, thighs and ankles, which had been present for 4 years and for which

FIGURE 2.1. Course of scratching in a case of neurodermatitis treated by a token economy procedure

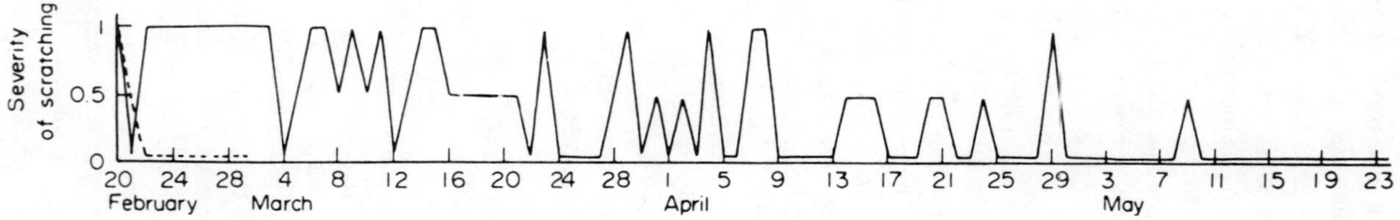

Scratching: 1, heavy; 0.5, slight; 0, nil; ——, night; ----, day.

he had been admitted to the clinic three times, without any lasting result. According to the patient the scratching had originally developed as a result of pruritus ani due to terminal ileitis. From the psychological examination the patient emerged as a rigid, tense personality, who could only with great difficulty cope with interpersonal relationships and could not express his feelings adequately. Because of lack of motivation and insight he did not appear to be accessible to verbal psychotherapy. Therefore we set up the following aversion procedure. The patient was seen once a day for a 20 min. session. He was instructed to bring his hand to his scrotum, upper leg or ankle to scratch at a sign from the therapist.

This sign was given every fifteen s.* At the moment his hand reached one of these sites, he received an unpleasant, though not painful, electric shock via electrodes on the fingers of the moving hand. He then had to draw back his hand and say aloud, "Don't scratch." In each session he received seventy-six shocks. He was also trained in relaxation exercises. After 19 days of treatment the scratching had disappeared completely and there was a consequent improvement in the skin disorder (Figure 2.2). Follow-up after 13 months showed that he had suffered three short, severe attacks of itching during which he could not refrain from scratching. After the end of such an attack there was no further scratching. In conditioning terms, punishing the neurotic behavior resulted in deconditioning the undesired and maladaptive habit.

Trichotillomania

Other forms of compulsive behaviour are the plucking of hairs from the head and eyebrows (trichotillomania), the production of dermatological artifacts and self-mutilation of the nails. Here too it is important to carry out an accurate psychosocial investigation. As with compulsive scratching it may be that existing emotional problems are not the cause of the undesired behaviour, but can be understood as a consequence of, or as a condition for, the maintainance of this behaviour which has begun to have an autonomous existence.

Taylor (1963) describes the treatment of a case of obsessive, compulsive eyebrow plucking and states that "since the emotional concomitants of the behaviour are a consequence of social criticism, which in turn is a consequence of the compulsive action, it is evident that any attempt to deal with the emotion must fail," and "our theory leads to the conclusion that the primary habit is likely to be the simplest component of the whole behavioural complex, and therefore most amenable to treatment." The patient described was a

---

*It appeared from further experience that administering the shock every 5s was equally effective.

FIGURE 2.2. Course of scratching in a case of neurodermatitis treated by shock-aversion therapy

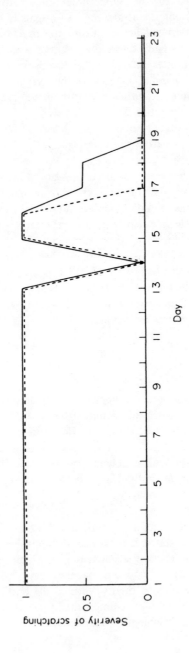

Scratching: 1, heavy; 0.5, slight; 0, nil; —— night; ----, day.

woman aged 40, who had been plucking her eyebrows compulsively for 31 years. She was instructed to stop at its commencement any movement of her hands to her forehead for the purpose of plucking. Cure was essentially complete in 10 days and 3 months later the eyebrows were fully grown. The rationale suggested by the author for this method was that "every time the impulse arose the patient was aware of it, not merely as an impulse to raise the hand to the forehead but as an impulse to pluck; and by preventing the initial response from progressing beyond the first millimetre she was in fact breaking down the whole response sequence."

There are patients, however, in whom the plucking of hairs is more or less unconscious. An instruction as given by Taylor is not sufficient in such cases. These patients have to be made aware that they are committing the unwanted activity. With the help of aversion therapy, as is described for scratching, the plucking or pulling appears to be rather rapidly brought under control. In the process of becoming more conscious, cognitive factors certainly play some significant role.

Case 3. A boy aged 14 had shown symptoms of trichotillomania for 1½ years. He had developed the habit of pulling out his hair, especially whilst he was reading or studying. A psychological investigation gave no indication of emotional problems. Pulling of his hair turned out to have a sensual significance for him. He reported that he knew that he pulled out his hair, but that he was not aware when he was actually doing it. The treatment consisted in breaking down the vicious circle by means of aversion therapy. In a period of 14 days he was able to refrain from this habit. He felt himself to have gained esteem from the people in his environment and he reported increased self-confidence. 2 months later there was some sporadic hair pulling, but after several "booster" sessions these residual symptoms totally disappeared. One of the disadvantages of aversion therapy is that it cannot always prevent a slight relapse into the old habits which can become very rewarding for the unwanted behaviour. Therefore, we advise some "booster" sessions if necessary.

Blushing

Not infrequently the dermatologist is confronted with patients who complain about chronic blushing. Psychological examination of these patients often shows that they are timid and inhibited in social contacts and situations. They dare not express their feelings, for fear of disapproval from others, so that they bottle up their emotions and begin to feel inferior. In social situations these patients react with autonomic vasomotor responses, including those in the face (symptomatic erythema), as an expression of their inhibited but conscious fears.

Based upon their social fear, which expresses itself in symptomatic erythema, a second form of fear often develops, namely the fear of becoming red (erythrophobia). Not infrequently the same kind of erythrophobia develops on the basis of an existing redness as in eczema or rosacea. So there is a second conditioning process in which the erythrophobia becomes an emotional response, which according to the classical conditioning paradigm, is elicited by the threatening situation and the symptomatic erythema connected to it. Gibbs (1965) states: "The blushing exacerbates the anxiety in a secondary way since the symptom itself embarrasses the patient." Since in these cases the inhibition of the ability to express emotions is the basic problem, the therapy will have to be directed towards learning to experience, accept and to express the inhibited emotions, such as anger, discontent, aggression, friendliness or affection, towards other people. Instead of escaping from the situation (e.g., by not expressing emotions) one trains the patient to behave more frankly in the face of the rising fear and thus to overcome it.

This method is called *assertive training* (Salter, 1950; Wolpe & Lazarus, 1966; Lazarus, 1971) and is based on Wolpe's theory of reciprocal inhibition (Wolpe, 1958). Assertive methods of training include amongst others: learning to express spontaneous feelings; learning to express one's own opinion clearly; learning to accept acknowledgments and praise; learning to cope with certain threatening situations, with the help of acting or role playing (behavioural rehearsal), where the therapist reinforces new, appropriate responses by praising them systematically. The theoretical background is that this form of behaviour will be strengthened in daily life by its positive consequences.

Salter, who was the designer of assertive training, described a case of chronic blushing in a patient with emotional inhibition phenomena and social fear (Salter, 1950, case 10). It is remarkable that, before the patient was instructed in his "six techniques for increasing excitation" the author instructed him to try to blush as much as possible in all kinds of situations and places. Within a week the patient appeared to have completely brought the involuntary blushing under voluntary control. Gibbs (1965) describes the treatment of a case of symptomatic erythema. The subject had been seriously troubled by excessive blushing in social situations for the previous 7 years. He was a man who constantly smiled, even under strong provocation. His embarrassment and blushing were greatest in personal contacts with his superiors in the hierarchy with whom he never disagreed. He frequently felt an impulse to be aggressive, but always inhibited its expression. Gibbs postulated that the symptoms were a learned response to anxiety. Treatment involved training in assertiveness. Considerable reduction in the frequency of blushing, together with improved social competence, were the results; the improvement was maintained over a follow-up period of 6 months.

Case 4. A student aged 22 with chronic constitutional eczema had also suffered from a symptomatic erythema for 4 years. The patient was descended from a narrow-minded, petit-bourgeois milieu, which he had outgrown by his studies and in which he felt out of place. The chronic blushing developed when he started studying in a foreign city. He was tormented by deep feelings of inferiority and uncertainty, which, strengthened by his existing skin disorder, handicapped normal social contacts until he retreated into almost complete solitude. With the help of the school doctor the worst phenomena of social fear were conquered, but after that he reacted to less subjective social threats by blushing with increased redness of his already red face, as a result of which the fear of blushing increased systematically. We attempted to break through this vicious circle by means of assertive training. The patient was advised to try to blush in as many situations as possible. After 5 days the blushing did not appear anymore. The feelings which assailed the patient in social situations, but which he tried to "suppress" spasmodically, were discussed and were thus experienced and accepted. During this process the therapist handled his approving remarks as operant reinforcers. Eventually the patient was taught to express his emotions, and also shown how he could make headway against socially threatening situations and thus overcome his fear. The social anxiety and fear of blushing disappeared rather rapidly and made room for a gradually strengthening feeling of self-confidence and skill in coping with interpersonal situations. 6 months later a check up showed not only no recurrence or symptom substitution, but also a continuously increasing ability to express himself adequately in social situations.

Although social fear is one of the most important characteristics of chronic blushing* this is not always determined by, or based upon, a lack of assertiveness. With accurate examination the existence of a phobia can sometimes be revealed in regard to certain specific aspects or objects in the environment. As Wolpe (1969) states: "Frequently fear and avoidance of social situations turn out to be based in fear of criticism or of rejection; or the fear may be a function of the mere physical presence of people, varying with the number to whom the patient is exposed." In these cases another therapeutic strategy must be applied to decondition the phobia; as for instance *systematic desensitization.*

Hyperhidrosis

Certain psychic reactions, like terror, fear, fury and strong concentration, are attended by increased sweating (Kuno, 1956). The palms and soles sweat more than normally in difficult life-situations and during psychic stress. Many people react even to small emotional stimuli with hyperhidrosis. This can give rise to secondary skin damage. Possibly a congenital form of hyperhidrosis also

---

*In many patients with urticaria there are not infrequently social fear, inhibition of feelings and a lack of assertiveness. In these cases assertive training can often be successfully used.

exists. This disorder can develop too as a result of contact hypersensitivity to certain substances.

Many patients with hyperhidrosis are afraid and not able to express their emotions. They can moreover become involved in a sort of vicious circle; the excessive perspiration or the fear of starting to sweat is sufficient to strengthen the fear and with that the hyperhidrosis (sudophobia). Some patients are not aware of this underlying fear, i.e., they only realize that they become frightened in a social situation, because someone may find out that they have wet hands. Psychological examination of these patients shows hypersensitive, restless, tense or frightened people. One can treat a number of these patients with sedatives and psychotherapeutic treatments. In patients who have repressed their fear very deeply the motivation for psychotherapeutic treatment is often absent. It is therapeutically sensible in these cases to provide help in breaking through the fear of social situations. *Assertive training* can produce good results here; i.e. the patient is taught to conquer fear reactions in interpersonal situations. *Systematic desensitization* can also be a good adjunct to the treatment.

Case 5. A girl aged 19 attended the dermatology out-patient clinic because of her severe palmar hyperhidrosis, present for some years and interfering with her work. She appeared to be in particularly great need of personal interest. As a child she felt that she was rapidly excluded by other people. She was also brought up with the idea that she had to do everything very well. She gradually developed strong feelings of insecurity when the environment did not regularly express positive appreciation of her. Moreover, she was not able to express her "negative" feelings. Her skin disorder became an extra reinforcement for her insecurity. The mere thought of having to shake hands with somebody produced an outburst of sweating. So it is possible that the sweating had become a conditioned reaction of fear for threatening stimuli (social situations). The normal sweat reaction to psychogenic stimuli, which was practically continuously active because of her insecurity and fear, was further reinforced by her fear of this reaction.

Through assertive training and systematic desensitization it became possible for the patient to feel more secure in social situations, to which her skin disorder reacted positively. Although the sweat gland activity was not completely "normal" even after some weeks, the patient was content with the improvement. A follow-up after 12 months showed no return to her old behaviour pattern.

We are now developing techniques in which, along with the above mentioned therapeutic methods, an attempt is made to condition instrumentally the sweat gland activity itself (Kuypers & Cotton, 1972).

Phobias

In those cases characterized by a fear of certain objects, situations or diseases, like syphilophobia or cancerophobia, perhaps *systematic desensitization* could be used. Case studies have not yet been published and our own experience with behaviour therapy of patients of this type is at the moment insufficient for a definite conclusion.

REFERENCES

Allen, K. & Harris, F. (1966) Elimination of a child's excessive scratching by training the mother in reinforcement procedures. *Behaviour Research and Therapy, 4*, 79.

Bandura, A. (1969) *Principles of Behaviour Modification.* Holt, Rinehart & Winston, London.

Gibbs, D. (1965) Reciprocal inhibition therapy of a case of symptomatic erythema. *Behaviour Research and Therapy, 3*, 261.

Kuno, Y. (1956) *Human perspiration.* Charles C. Thomas, Springfield, Ill.

Kuypers, B. & Cotton, D. (1972) Conditioning of sweating. A preliminary report. *British Journal of Dermatology, 87*, 154.

Lazarus, A. (1971) *Behaviour Therapy and Beyond.* McGraw-Hill, New York.

Ratliff, R. & Stein, N. (1968) Treatment of neurodermatitis by behaviour therapy: a case study. *Behaviour Research and Therapy, 6*, 397.

Salter, A. (1950) *Conditioned Reflex Therapy.* Creative Age Press, New York.

Taylor, J. (1963) A behavioural interpretation of obsessive-compulsive neurosis. *Behaviour Research and Therapy, 1*, 237.

Walton, D. (1960) The application of learning theory to the treatment of a case of neuro-dermatitis. In: *Behavior Therapy and the Neuroses* (Ed. by H. J. Eysenck), p. 272. Pergamon Press, Oxford.

Wolpe, J. (1958) *Psychotherapy by Reciprocal Inhibition.* Stanford University Press.

Wolpe, J. (1969) *The Practice of Behavior Therapy.* Pergamon Press, New York.

Wolpe, J. & Lazarus, A. (1966) *Behaviour Therapy Techniques.* Pergamon Press, Oxford.

Yates, A. (1970) *Behavior Therapy.* Wiley & Sons, New York.

MANAGEMENT OF MALADAPTIVE BEHAVIOR
OF A SEVERELY BURNED CHILD

Clayton T. Shorkey
John E. Taylor

Management of learning experiences that contribute to emotional problems of severely injured children requires considerable attention by workers in the medical area. Behavior-modification theory provides a useful framework for the assessment and management of such problems. The following case involving a severely burned child illustrates the use of behavior-modification techniques.

Physical damage and painful treatment procedures often produce anxiety and panic reactions, as well as aggressive and regressive behavior, in children suffering severe burns.(6) Undesirable behavior hinders or in some cases prevents successful medical treatment.(2) Repeated unsuccessful attempts by staff members to deal with such behaviors often result in staff fatigue, feelings of helplessness and frequent transfer of nurses to other medical units.(3)

A major source of the development of maladaptive emotional behavior is an increase in pain or discomfort to the child because of the injury or the medical treatment. A second source of problems is the child's inability to achieve customary positive reinforcement.

Increased pain or discomfort provides the stimuli for learning escape or avoidance behaviors, classically conditioned anxiety responses to the treatment, and pervasive anxiety. Any aspect of the treatment may become associated

Reprinted from *Child Welfare*, 1973, *52*, 543-547. Copyright 1973 by Child Welfare. Reprinted by permission.

Clayton T. Shorkey, M.S.W., Ph.D., is associate professor, School of Social Work, University of Texas at Austin. John E. Taylor, M.S.W., is assistant program director, Atascadero State Hospital, Atascadero, California.

with pain or discomfort and take on aversive characteristics. Through association with aversive stimuli, many aspects of the child's world may become formidable and threatening. In most situations little relief is available to counteract the aversive developments.

Injuries and painful medical treatment may also reduce the child's ability to carry out habitual patterns of behavior previously effective in achieving reinforcement. The child may be unable to exercise his body freely and to behave in ways that are in themselves a source of reinforcement.(5) Reduction in the ability to achieve customary reinforcements can result in frustration and aggression in the form of intrapunitive and extrapunitive behavior. Frustration may also result in regression or a return to patterns of behaviors that earlier were effective in achieving reinforcement.(4) Depression, also related to the lessened ability of the individual to achieve customary reinforcement, is particularly prevalent with individuals suffering severe physical damage. Such changes in the client's arousal level may reduce overall motivation to participate in the treatment process.(7) Each of these problems—frustration, aggression, regression and depression—may be minimized by providing the opportunity for the individual to achieve reinforcement for behaviors that approximate those required for readjustment.

Although neither increased aversive stimuli nor reduced ability to achieve customary reinforcement can be eliminated by the use of behavior-modification techniques, learning experiences may be controlled to reduce maladaptive behaviors. The following case illustrates the assessment and behavior management of severely maladaptive behavior of a burned child.

CASE HISTORY

The patient was a 17-month-old girl suffering from second- and third-degree burns on 37% of her body, involving both legs, the perineum, buttocks and both hands and wrists. The baby was placed in isolation on admission to the hospital. She was quiet during admission but cried frequently during the next few days. The child cried lustily and moved her limbs in an agitated way when the nurses squirted silver nitrate over the bandages. The nurses attempted to console her at such times. After 4 weeks of this regime, the nursing staff recorded that the baby was refusing food and became extremely agitated when approached by a staff member. Her physical condition deteriorated and skin grafts were discontinued.

At this point the hospital social worker was called in. The worker observed that the nurses, who were extremely disturbed at the child's condition, would interrupt the treatment and spend much time attempting to soothe the child by talking to her, singing and playing with her toys. Such activity had no effect on the crying or apparent high anxiety. Also, the nurses would frequently visit the child in an attempt to talk to her or play with her between treatments. The entrance of a staff member evoked agitation and loud crying and caused the baby to try to look away from the staff member. This behavior was hindered because the child was kept in restraints to avoid self-injury by body agitation.

Systematic observations indicated that the staff members had become conditioned aversive stimuli through their association with the painful treatment and that their entrance and continual presence in the room were evoking strong undesirable responses. This situation was complicated by the baby's total inability to speak or to avoid the aversive aspects of her environment because of restraints.

Observation by the worker of the feeding procedure indicated that the child could not comfortably swallow the amount of food presented in the spoon. The child displayed anxiety during feeding and attempted to avoid the food. When a spoonful of food was placed in her mouth, she often would choke and spit it out. This feeding procedure increased the anxiety reaction of the child to the staff members. The process of eating is extremely sensitive to suppression through aversive stimuli.(1) Therefore, a corrected procedure of feeding was considered extremely important in this case.

PROCEDURES

A system of behavior management was developed by the social worker and nurses in an attempt to counteract previous learning of the child in the hospital and to confine her distress to treatment periods. The first step was designed to teach the child to discriminate between aversive conditions (medical treatment) and nonaversive conditions (social interactions).

As to treatment, the nurses continued to wear green isolation gowns, but were instructed not to talk to the child, handle her unnecessarily, play with her toys or spend unnecessary time in the room. Treatments were carried out with the white room lights turned on. This was done to identify the treatment situation clearly and to avoid further association of the voices of staff, toys, etc., with the aversive stimuli of the medical treatment.

As to social conditions, staff members wore red, sterilized bags with armholes when entering the room to play with the child. Red flood lights installed in the room were operated at these times. Also, the staff members spent a brief time massaging the infant's neck and top of her shoulders, which had not been burned, to reduce the muscle tenseness that arose because she was restrained on the bed on her stomach. The massaging was an attempt to produce relaxation and thus reduce anxiety.

The second part of the behavior-management procedure involved the feeding process. The nurses fed the child after massaging her neck and shoulders. They offered small amounts of food on their fingers, rather than using utensils, and were instructed to carry out the procedure in a slow and relaxed way. The plan called for reinstatement of the use of utensils after the child began to eat regularly.

MOTHER'S REACTIONS

The child's mother at first refused to cooperate with the staff in the procedures, since she believed that the child would be calmed by the child's eventual recognition of her as mother. Because the child continued to react to the mother in the same way as to the staff members, the social worker gave the mother a red apron instead of a plastic bag, thus differentiating the mother from the staff, but maintaining the discrimination between social and treatment procedures.

Consistent use of discrimination and counterconditioning procedures decreased the child's anxiety responses under the social condition and reduced the number of times that the infant became upset during the brief treatment periods every 2 hours. Changes in the child's behavior were not observed until the second day of the regime. At that time, crying lessened during the social period and the child began to watch silently as staff members entered her room. Two days later the child smiled during this period for the first time. By the fourth day the staff began to induce smiling by playing a peek-a-boo game, and by the end of the 2 weeks the child appeared comfortable and smiled during these visits. Behavior during treatment remained unchanged.

The infant's ability to differentiate between treatment and feeding procedures allowed resumption of skin grafting.

The discrimination procedures were continued for 1½ months until the child was in relatively good physical condition, showed little fear of hospital personnel and ate satisfactorily. The last weeks of hospitalization were relatively painless and the discrimination procedure was dropped 2 weeks before the child was released.

The use of the behavior-modification techniques in this case not only produced changes in the behavior of the child that allowed treatment to be resumed, but was a source of reinforcement for the staff.

Followup information for up to 2 years indicated that there were no detectable problems in physical recovery or psychological problems associated with the injury or treatment. The child had been placed in the care of her grandmother after release, because the mother indicated that the injury might not have been accidental, and expressed fear that other such incidents might occur if she maintained the child.

CONCLUSIONS

The authors believe that the use of behavior-modification techniques in the management of social and emotional behavior of children being treated for severe illness or injury should be given more attention by professionals in medical settings. Use of such techniques requires an assessment of each case through careful observation and the formulation of procedures that meet the needs of the individual client.

REFERENCES

1. Bandura, A. "Presentation of Negative Reinforcers," in Principles of Behavior Modification. New York: Holt, Rinehart and Winston, 1969.
2. Craig, R. D. P. "Survival From Extensive Burns in Childhood," British Journal of Surgery, LIII (1966).
3. Long, R. T., and Cope, O. "Emotional Problems of Burned Children," New England Journal of Medicine, CCLXIV (1961).
4. Lundin, R W. "Frustration and Conflict 1," in Personality: A Behavioral Analysis. London: Macmillan, 1969.
5. Premock, D. "Toward Empirical Behavior Laws 1: Positive Reinforcement," Psychological Review, LXVI (1959).
6. Stoll, C. P. "Responses of Three Girls to Burn Injuries and Hospitalization," Nursing Clinics of North America, IV (1969).
7. Ullmann, L. P., and Krasner, L. "Affective Reactions and Suicide," in A Psychological Approach to Abnormal Behavior, Englewood Cliffs, N.J.: Prentice-Hall, 1969.

3

DENTISTRY

INTRODUCTION

Pedodontists need exceptional behavioral management skills. They must gain the trust and confidence of their young patients and simultaneously allay the parents' anxieties. Children coming to dentists generally have not been adequately prepared to have had a prior aversive experience. Too often children coming for treatment bring their parents' dental anxieties with them. Pedodontists are now providing pretreatment visits to their clinics to familiarize children with their offices, dental personnel, and equipment. This procedure, if used correctly, can provide an opportunity for desensitization of normal anxieties, as well as provide some inoculation against development of dental fears.

During treatment, children must consent to enter the operatory and sit in the dental chair, open their mouths on command, and submit to examination. Further they must accept injections and the resulting deadening, as well as the various sensations of mechanical operations in the mouth, including drilling, abrading, and polishing. In the case of children who have already experienced previous dental traumas, merely getting these battleworn veterans back into the dental office may be an outstanding feat. If children have successfully avoided treatment by throwing tantrums, crying, or fainting, it may be doubly difficult to get them into the treatment area. If children successfully avoid dental care, the resulting phobia can easily generalize to other medical treatment settings.

The application of behavioral techniques for dealing with common dental problems of children may be classified into three areas: contingency management, desensitization, and vicarious symbolic modeling. Contingency management procedures have increased dental adherence behaviors such as sitting quietly in the chair, keeping the hands in the lap, opening and keeping the mouth open on command, and other cooperative behaviors necessary for effective treatment (Kimmelman, 1964; Kohlenberg, Greenberg, Reymore, & Hass, 1972; Rosenberg, 1974). Desensitization has been used along with modeling procedures to explore the relative effectiveness of the two procedures. Adelson and Goldfried (1970), in their article included in this section, entitled "Modeling and the Fearful Child Patient," were innovative in the use of systematic desensitization and emotive imagery to deal with dental phobias. Additionally, the authors used observation of a nonfearful person modeling appropriate dental behaviors. They advocate the use of either live or filmed models and suggest that the modeling presented by the dentist and staff are also crucial to children's responses to their first and subsequent dental appointments. Machen and Johnson (1974) and Gordon, Terdal and Sterling (1974) present other studies combining the use of these techniques in the treatment of dental phobias. Modeling with preschool children was shown to be effective in curtailing phobic behavior in young patients (White, Akers, Green & Yates, 1974). Approach and avoidance behavior checklists were presented, breaking down behaviors into useful categories. Children received instruction and "treatment" for toothbrushing, oral examination, prophylaxis fluoride treatment, injection, and a restorative procedure.

In a series of studies, Melamed and associates (Melamed, Hawes, Heiby, & Glick, 1975; Melamed, Weinstein, Hawes & Katin-Borland, 1975; Melamed, Yurcheson, Fleece, Hutcherson, & Hawes, 1978) have systematically explored the use of modeling through film presentations to increase cooperativeness in young patients. Sawtell, Simon, and Simeonsson (1974), in contrast to the findings of Machen and Johnson (1974), found no differences between desensitization and modeling. Melamed et al. (1978), in a study of 80 children undergoing three dental sessions involving prophylaxis, dental examination, and dental restorative treatment, found that age and previous experience of the viewer were important in determining children's responses to vicarious peer modeling. Though it is clear from this and other related studies that systematic desensitization and modeling procedures cannot be used with equal effectiveness with all patients, under all dental conditions, one is made aware of the complexities of dealing with such problems. Perhaps in no other area reviewed in this book has modeling been applied so consistently and creatively in attempting to deal with children's anxieties.

Recognizing the importance of good management skills in the treatment of children's dental problems, the pediatric dentistry journals, such as *The Journal of Dentistry for Children*, regularly carry articles dealing with improving these skills. One especially difficult problem faced by dentists is the management of developmentally handicapped children, especially those who are mentally retarded. Kohlenberg, Greenberg, Reymore, and Hass (1972) reviewed a number of operant techniques that can be used by dentists who treat retarded children. More recently, Troutman (1977) presented an excellent review of the special dental requirements of mentally retarded children. He offered a number of alternatives to more coercive dental techniques, such as the "tell-show-do" technique to orient children to the dental setting, and the use of various behavioral approaches for treatment.

In his article on pediatric dentistry with handicapped children, included in this chapter, Drash (1971) reviewed behavioral techniques with both retarded and emotionally disturbed children. Principles of behavioral change and techniques for producing change are discussed in light of the problems experienced by dentists. This article is particularly valuable in its demonstration of how simple behavior techniques can be applied to perennial dental management problems.

Nineteen percent of the American child population are true dental phobics (Keys, 1978). A number of researchers have speculated on the etiology, assessment, and treatment of the phobia (for example, Marks, 1978; Sermet, 1974; Keys, 1978; Keys, Field, & Korboot, 1978). Several methods, such as the Corah Dental Anxiety Scale (Corah, 1969) can be used to assess anxiety in dental patients. Johnson and Machen (1973) and Wright, Alpern, and Leake (1973) discussed the role of maternal anxieties in the development and maintenance of dental phobias in children. Hill and O'Mullane (1976), in a very practical article, outline a four-visit program to prevent these anxieties. Similarly, Ayer (1973) described the use of visual imagery to eliminate needle phobia in children. Several writers have suggested the use of the tell-show-do procedure (Howitt & Stricker, 1965) mentioned earlier, wherein the dentist will, over several sessions, tell children about each preparation and procedure that they will experience, and show them the equipment and procedures before treating them. Informal relaxation procedures along with the tell-show-do procedure are also used.

Chambers (1977) argues that there is no shortage of techniques for managing children in the dental office and suggests that behavioral approaches represent one of the most useful resources. He argues that dentistry as a profession must develop a consensus on standards for appropriate dental behaviors of young children, adapt the pediatric dental curriculum so that students can learn how normal healthy children ought to behave in the dental chair, and develop a cumulative research literature that focuses on the need for providing dental care rather than a series of technique demonstrations.

References

Adelson, R., & Goldfried, M. R. Modeling and the fearful child patient. *ASDC Journal of Dentistry for Children*, 1970, *37*, 476-489.

Ayer, W. A. Use of visual imagery in needle phobic children. *ASDC Journal of Dentistry for Children*, 1973, *40*, 125-127.

Chambers, D. W. Behavior management techniques for pediatric dentists: An embarassment of riches. *ASDC Journal of Dentistry for Children*, 1977, *44*, 30-34.

Corah, N. L. Development of dental anxiety scale. *Journal of Dental Research*, 1969, *48*, 596.

Drash, P. W. Behavior modification: New tools for use in pediatric dentistry with the handicapped child. *Dental Clinics of North America*, 1971, *18*, 617-631.

Gordon, D. A., Terdal, L., & Sterling, E. Use of modeling and desensitization in the treatment of a phobic child patient. *ASDC Journal of Dentistry for Children*, 1974, *41*, 102-105.

Hill, F. J., & O'Mullane, D. M. A preventive program for the dental management of frightened children. *ASDC Journal of Dentistry for Children*, 1976, *43*, 326-330.

Howitt, J. W., & Stricker, G. Child patient responses to various dental procedures. *Journal of the American Dental Association*, 1965, *70*, 70-74.

Johnson, R., & Machen, J. B. Behavior modification techniques and maternal anxiety. *Journal of Dentistry for Children*, 1973, *40*, 272-276.

Keys, J. Detecting and treating dental phobic children: Part I, detection. *ASDC Journal of Dentistry for Children*, 1978, *45*, 296-300.

Keys, J., Field, M., & Korboot, P. Detecting and treating dental phobic children: Part II, treatment. *ASDC Journal of Dentistry for Children*, 1978, *45*, 301-305.

Kimmelman, B. B. Management of sensitive children in a general dental practice. *ASDC Journal of Dentistry for Children*, 1964, *31*, 146-150.

Kohlenberg, R., Greenberg, D., Reymore, L., & Hass, G. Behavior modification in the management of mentally retarded dental patients. *ASDC Journal of Dentistry for Children*, 1972, *39*, 61-67.

Machen, J. B., & Johnson, R. Desensitization, model learning, and the dental behavior of children. *Journal of Dental Research*, 1974, *53*, 83-87.

Marks, H. S. The genesis of fear and anxiety in young dental patients. *ASDC Journal of Dentistry for Children*, 1978, *45*, 306-309.

Melamed, B. G., Hawes, R. R., Heiby, E., & Glick, J. The use of film modeling to reduce uncooperative behavior of children during dental treatment. *Journal of Dental Research*, 1975, *54*, 797-801.

Melamed, B. G., Weinstein, D., Hawes, R., & Katin-Borland, M. Reduction of fear-related dental management using filmed modeling. *Journal of the American Dental Association*, 1975, *90*, 822-826.

Melamed, B. G., Yurcheson, R., Fleece, E. L., Hutcherson, S., & Hawes, R. Effects of film modeling on the reduction of anxiety-related behaviors in individuals varying in level of previous experience in the stress situation. *Journal of Consulting and Clinical Psychology*, 1978, *46*, 1357-1367.

Rosenberg, H. M. Behavior modification for the child dental patient. *ASDC Journal of Dentistry for Children*, 1974, *41*, 111-114.

Sawtell, R. O., Simon, J. F., & Simeonsson, R. J. Effects of five preparatory methods upon child behavior during the first dental visit. *ASDC Journal of Dentistry for Children*, 1974, *41*, 367-375.

Sermet, O. Emotional and medical factors in child dental anxiety. *Journal of Child Psychology and Psychiatry*, 1974, *15*, 313-321.

Troutman, K. Behavioral management of the mentally retarded. *Dental Clinics of North America*, 1977, *21*, 621-636.

White, W. C. Jr., Akers, J., Green, J., & Yates, D. Use of imitation in the treatment of dental phobia in early childhood: A preliminary report. *ASDC Journal of Dentistry for Children*, 1974, *41*, 106-110.

Wright, G. Z., Alpern, G. D., & Leake, J. L. The modifiability of maternal anxiety as it relates to children's cooperative dental behavior. *ASDC Journal of Dentistry for Children*, 1973, *40*, 265-271.

MODELING AND THE FEARFUL CHILD PATIENT

Richard Adelson
Marvin R. Goldfried

All dentists who treat children occasionally find themselves faced with the fearful child in his first visit to the dentist. Considering the awesomeness of dental equipment, and the newness of the experience, it is not surprising that the child may be apprehensive. In addition, it is not uncommon to find the child's fear exaggerated by the stories told by peers and siblings, and by the fears of the parents themselves.

Apart from making the examination and treatment procedures more difficult, or even impossible, the fear associated with dentistry may have long-term consequences as well. Early dental experiences will influence later attitudes. Frequently the adult patient refuses dental care because of the poor introduction he had to dentistry.

The great importance of the introduction of the child to dentistry is unquestioned. Much has been written on the subject. Suggestions include one or more of the following components: (1) a patient, understanding, and permissive doctor who is willing to spend numerous visits with the child until his dental office, the treatment room, and various treatment procedures are no longer new and frightening to the patient; (2) a "tell, show, do" procedure, whereby the child is told what will be done, shown what will be done, and

Reprinted from *Journal of Dentistry for Children*, 1970, *37*, 34-37. Copyright 1979 by American Society of Dentistry for Children. Reprinted by permission.

Richard Adelson, D.D.S., is associate professor of dental medicine, School of Dental Medicine, State University of New York at Stony Brook, and coordinator of medical and dental education, Veteran's Administration Northeast Regional Medical Education Center.

Marvin Goldfried, Ph.D. is professor of psychology, Department of Psychology, State University of New York at Stony Brook.

then treated; (3) the use of pre-medication, so that the patient may arrive at the treatment room in a more compliant state. [1-12] Although these methods have been found to result in a fair degree of success, they have some important drawbacks. The first method is inefficient and uneconomical. In addition, this technique requires a dentist who is very sensitive to the behavior and emotions of children, and knows the pace at which to proceed. The success of the "tell, show, do" procedure similarly depends upon a certain amount of psychological sensitivity and skill. More important, however, is the fact that research evidence indicates that although some success may be achieved with children who are only mildly anxious, it is not very effective with the highly anxious child. [13]

The inadequacy of these techniques has led to the use of drugs to assure patient control. Current literature notes some of the negative consequences of drug use, including the danger of overmedication and the potential idiosyncratic reaction to drugs. [2, 14, 15]

In looking for an effective and practical technique of dealing with the child's fear, let us turn to the field of psychology. To date psychological principles have been employed mainly in an attempt to understand the child's emotional development. [2, 14, 16, 17, 18] Changing behavior patterns, language development, and ability to learn at different age levels are some of the areas that have been discussed in the literature. Very little work, however, has been done by dentists to bring about reduction of anxiety in child patients.

Recent emphasis in the field of clinical psychology on "behavior modification" provides us with techniques which may be useful in dentistry. In addition to earlier suggestions for the use of *pleasurable activities* and *gradual habituation* in the elimination of children's fears, some of the more recent procedures with children have included the use of *systematic desensitization*— i.e., the gradual presentation of the feared stimulus while the person is under a state of relaxation, *emotive imagery*—i.e., the presentation in imagination of the feared situation in conjunction with some highly pleasant situation, and *modeling procedures*—i.e., the observation of a non-fearful child in the same situation. [19-23] It is the last of these procedures that we believe to be most relevant to the management of the apprehensive child patient.

Part of the basic philosophy underlying modeling techniques is that personality develops through an individual's social learning experiences. [24] Particularly during childhood, a good deal of the development and learning that goes on is based on the individual's imitation of others. By observing a model, a child is able to learn complex behavior patterns which would otherwise require much trial and error before they could be obtained. Learning through modeling is particularly effective when the observer is in a state of arousal, when the model has relatively more status and prestige, and when there are positive consequences of the model's behavior.

Modeling has proved effective for a number of uses. Included in these are the behavioral changes brought about in cooperation behavior, language development, moral judgments, self-rewarding responses, delay of gratification patterns, and reduction of fear.

The most relevant application to dentistry appears to be in the introduction of the child to a new, unstructured environment, and in the reduction of anxiety. Bandura and his associates have recently demonstrated in a controlled study that children's fear of dogs can be successfully reduced by means of modeling procedures.[23] After having the opportunity to observe a fearless model playing with a dog in a series of gradually increasing fear-provoking sessions, fearful nursery school children became less afraid themselves. The finding was later replicated with the use of a filmed model.[25]

CASE STUDY DEMONSTRATING THE USE OF MODELING

Although the effectiveness of modeling procedures in influencing and modifying behavior was recognized by the senior author, the application of modeling in the management of the apprehensive child was not implemented until two children were to make simultaneous visits to the office for examination. The two children, unrelated, were Amy (age four), and Penny (age three and one-half). Amy who was bold and friendly, with a prior pleasant dental experience, appeared to have little fear of a dental appointment. Penny, who had never been to the dentist before, was shy and withdrawn, and was obviously worried about what the dental examination would be like. Based on previous experience, a management problem was anticipated.

The decision was made to use Amy for a model, and Penny was invited into the treatment room to "just watch." Penny sat in the back of the room, where she could have a good view of the treatment procedure. The clinical examination conducted with Amy included mouth mirror and explorer, visual examination, radiographs, and soft tissue examination. As we expected, Amy was cheerful, responsive, and cooperative throughout the examination. She was told that since she was so cooperative, she was to receive a special prize, a ring which she could select from a small "treasure chest." In leaving the chair, Amy stood on the footstep for a moment and then jumped with both feet together, so that she landed with a loud "clump."

Amy left the room, and it was Penny's turn to be examined. Although still reticent, she was perfectly willing to get into the chair. Identical examination procedures were carried out with Penny. In contrast to what was expected with a child such as Penny, there were no management problems whatsoever. It was not until the examination was completed and Penny had received her "reward" that it was realized how greatly her behavior was influenced by the model. Penny went through the identical procedure in getting off the chair, landing on the floor with the same "clump."

Penny was seen six months later for a recall appointment which consisted of prophylaxis, polishing, and fluoride treatments. She was extremely cooperative. It is interesting to note at this later date that she got down from the chair the same way.

In analyzing the various components of this situation, we see that not only was the observer in a high state of arousal (worried and apprehensive), but the model represented someone of high status (slightly older, gregarious, and comfortable socially), and that there were positive consequences following the behavior (a ring was given as a reward to the model).

DISCUSSION AND CONCLUSIONS

As a result of previous research findings and case studies, it appears that the greatest value of modeling would be for the general practitioner in the introduction of children into his practice. The highly anxious, fearful child is least susceptible to those techniques which previously have been used to allay fears and instill confidence. Modeling procedures constitute an approach that requires a minimal amount of professional time and can easily become part of the dentist's office routine.

The use of modeling techniques should prove particularly effective in the clinic. In clinic situations where there are a large number of patients to be treated with limited personnel, we often find that the apprehensive child is poorly handled. The child's first visit, furthermore, is usually an emergency situation. The child often comes with pain and swelling, and his normal fears are exaggerated. He is usually examined, and then restrained physically so that treatment can be performed. Such initial experience virtually assures a traumatic future even when only minimal work is required. Following the work of Bandura and his associates on effects of vicarious experience, a film can be shown to new patients as they enter the clinic, giving them a favorable model undergoing and experiencing the procedure to be used.[23] We can produce then a less fearful and more compliant and cooperative patient. To quote Bandura, ". . . skillfully designed therapeutic films could be developed and employed in preventive programs for eliminating common fears and anxieties before they become well-established and widely generalized." [23]

The dentist is also acting as a model, and his behavior will have a great effect on the behavior of his patient. The doctor who is calm, relaxed, confident, and positive is more likely to produce similar reactions in the patient. On the other hand, the dentist who is upset, anxious, and nervous, is likely to heighten the anxiety and nervousness of the patient. The use of modeling is particularly relevant in the introduction of patients to the use of analgesia, especially since research findings have demonstrated that individuals who exhibit similar physiological responses can, depending upon the behavior of a model, experience different emotional reactions.[26] Thus, actually seeing another person—*in vivo* or by way of a film—react favorably to analgesia, is likely to produce a positive patient response.

Many dentists are missing the rewards of treating children. It is because of unpleasant experiences with the fearful child that some dentists refuse to treat children. We have presented here a method that is both effective and efficient. It will reach the child for whom other methods have proved of little value, and just as important, it will produce results in a fraction of the time otherwise necessary.

BIBLIOGRAPHY

1. Kimmelman, Benedict B.: Management of Sensitive Children in a General Dental Practice. *J Dent Child, 31*:146-150, 2nd qtr., 1964.
2. Olsen, Norman H.: Behavior Control of the Child Dental Patient. *J Amer Dent Assoc, 68*:873-877, June, 1964.
3. Dov, Laufer; Rosenzweig, Kurt A.; and Chosak, Aubrey: Explanation as a Means of Reducing Fear of Dental Procedures in Children, *Alpha Omegan, 56*:130-133, September, 1964.
4. Cherches, Mark L. and Blackman, Sheldon: Alleviating the Anxiety of Children in Dental Treatment. *J Amer Dent Assoc, 66*:824-826, June, 1963.
5. Finn, Sidney B. and others: *Clinical pedodontics*, Ch. 2-3, Philadelphia, W. B. Saunders, 1957.
6. Buckman, Norman: Balanced Premedication with Pedodontics. *Dent Abstr, 4:5*, January, 1959.
7. Lampshire, Earl L.: Balanced Medication—an Aid for the Child Patient. *Dent Clin N Amer*, 507-519, November, 1961.
8. Anderson, Jack L.: Use of Chloral Hydrate in Dentistry. *Northwest Dent, 39*:33-35, January, 1960.
9. Stetson, John B. and Jessup, Gretchen: Use of Chloral Hydrate Mixtures for Pediatric Premedication. Anesthesia and Analgesia. . . *Current Researches, 41*:203-215, March-April, 1962.
10. Lang, Larry L.: An Evaluation of the Efficacy of Using Hydroxyzine in Controlling the Behavior of Child Patients. *J Dent Child, 32*: 253-258, October, 1965.
11. Stewart, Joseph G.: Routine Preoperative Medication in Dentistry for Children. *J Dent Child, 28*:209-212, 3rd qtr., 1961.
12. Peabody, Joseph B.: Premedicating Pedodontic Patients. *Texas Dent J, 83*:10:12-15, October, 1965.
13. Howitt, Jack W. and Stricker, George: Child response to various procedures. *J Amer Dent Assoc, 70*:70-74, January, 1965.
14. Garfin, Laurence A.: Factors in the Management of the Child Patient. *J Dent Child, 39*:179-184, 3rd. qtr., 1962.

15. Anderson, Robert H.: Dangers of Premedication. *J Calif Dent Assoc and the Official Organ of the Nevada Dent Soc, 36*:367-373, October, 1960.
16. Aduss, Howard; Bane, Rodney S.; and Lang, Larry L.: Pedodontic Psychology and Premedication. *J Dent Child, 28*:73-83, 1st qtr., 1961.
17. Massler, Maury: Psychology in Dentistry for Children. *Dent Clin N Amer*, 623-635, November, 1962.
18. Kleiser, John R. Application of psychological principles to dental practice.
17. Massler, Maury: Psychology in Dentistry for Children. *Dent Clin N Amer* 623-635, November, 1962.
18. Kleiser, John R.: Application of psychological principles to dental practice. *J Dent Child, 33*:113-117, March, 1966.
19. Jones, Mary C.: The elimination of children's fears. *J Exp Psychol, 7*: 382-390, October, 1924.
20. Jersild, Arthur T. and Holmes, Frances B.: Methods of overcoming children's fears. *J Psychol, L*:75-104, first half, 1935.
21. Lazarus, Arnold A.: The elimination of children's phobias by deconditioning. In Eysenck, Hans J. (Ed.) *Experiments in behavior therapy.* New York: MacMillan Company, 1964.
22. Lazarus, Arnold A. and Abramovitz, Arnold: The Use of "Emotive Imagery" in the Treatment of Children's Phobias. *J Ment Sci, 108*: 191-195, March, 1962.
23. Bandura, Albert; Grusec, Joan E.; and Menlove, Frances L.: Vicarious extinction of avoidance behavior. *J Personality Soc Psychol, 5*: 16-23, January, 1967.
24. Bandura, Albert and Walters, Richard H.: *Social Learning and Personality Development.* New York: Holt, Rinehart and Winston, 1963.
25. Bandura, Albert and Menlove, Frances L: Factors determining vicarious extinction of avoidance behavior through symbolic modeling. *J Personality Soc Psychol, 8*:99-108, February, 1968.
26. Schachter, Stanley and Singer, Jerome E.: Cognitive, Social and Physiological Determinants of Emotional States. *Psychol Rev, 69*:379-399, September, 1962.

BEHAVIOR MODIFICATION:
NEW TOOLS FOR USE
IN PEDIATRIC DENTISTRY
WITH THE HANDICAPPED CHILD

Philip W. Drash

One of the recurrent problems encountered by the pedodontist who deals with the handicapped child is that of obtaining the patient's cooperation while engaging in various dental procedures which will be of ultimate benefit to the child. Behavior control, including the elimination of anxiety and fear responses, is of obvious importance in general pediatric dentistry, and has been the subject of several recent investigations. [1, 5, 6, 8]

[11] The problem of behavior control is magnified many times over in the case of the mentally handicapped child who often does not understand the significance of the dental procedures and who may, in fact, have limited language comprehension so that verbal explanations and reassurances, which might be effective with the normal child, may have little or no controlling effect upon the behavior of the mentally handicapped child. [9] In the case of the emotionally disturbed child, the problem may be further compounded by the presence of severe temper tantrums, explosive and unpredictable outbursts, aggressive or destructive behavior, or at the opposite extreme, almost total withdrawal and consequent refusal to cooperate.

In the past, the pediatric dentist, when faced with an uncooperative, aggressive, or extremely anxious and withdrawn child, has had few options other than physical restraint, sedation, or general anesthesia.

Reprinted from *Dental Clinics of North America*, 1974, 18, 617-31. Copyright 1974 by W. B. Saunders Publications. Reprinted with permission.

Philip W. Drash, Ph.D., is professor and director of the Child Adolescent and Community Programs, Florida Mental Health Institute, Tampa, Florida. This work was supported in part by Grant No 917 Maternal and Child Health Services, U.S. Department of Health, Education, and Welfare to the Johns Hopkins University School of Medicine.

Within recent years, however, the science and technology of behavior control have made rapid advances[3] and there is now available to the pediatric dentist, a set of specific behavior modification procedures,[2, 4, 10] some of which can be automated in the dental office. These procedures will often allow him to increase vastly the precision and degree of control he is able to exert over the behavior of his patients. While the pedodontist is often the person called upon to treat the handicapped child, and therefore profit by the use of behavior modification, this technique should by no means be limited to use by pedodontists and only with the handicapped. It behooves all dentists to become familiar with the basic principles of behavior modification, and skilled in the technology of the control of human behavior.

BASIC PRINCIPLES OF BEHAVIOR CONTROL

Behavior as a Function of Its Consequences

Contrary to popular opinion, which places the locus of behavior control in those stimulus events which precede the behavior, most complex human behavior is, in fact, shaped, maintained, controlled, or eliminated as a direct function or consequence of those stimulus events which immediately follow the behavior. Thus, for example, if a child begins crying upon being placed in the dental chair, the crying is most productively viewed, from the standpoint of behavior control, not as a fear response elicited by the sight of the dental chair and equipment, i.e., stimuli preceding the behavior, but by the fact that in similar situations, crying has been reinforced or rewarded by removal from the dental chair and avoidance of dental work, i.e., consequences of the behavior.

Positive and Negative Reinforcers

Based upon their behavioral effects, stimuli may be classified into three categories, namely, positive reinforcers, aversive stimuli, and neutral stimuli.

Positive Reinforcers. A positive reinforcer is operationally defined as any stimulus event which will increase the frequency of a behavior or a response which it immediately follows. Those stimuli which have survival value for the organism such as food and water usually serve as positive reinforcers. In addition, there are a large number of social and environmental stimuli which have acquired reinforcing properties, such as a smile, a word of praise, a compliment, a touch, or various environmental stimuli such as toys, cosmetics, and other personal possessions, or engaging in a wide variety of activities which are generally considered pleasurable. Since a reinforcer is operationally defined by its ability to increase the frequency of a response, it is obvious that a stimulus which may serve as a reinforcer for one child may not serve as a reinforcer for another. Furthermore, a stimulus which may serve as a reinforcer for a child on one occasion may not serve as a reinforcer for the same child at some later time.

Aversive Stimuli. An aversive stimulus may be defined either as a stimulus which will decrease the frequency of a behavior which it immediately follows or as a stimulus which will increase the frequency of any response which terminates or reduces the intensity of the stimulus. While the former definition is somewhat more straightforward, the latter is more sensitive and more functional in that a relatively mild stimulus, such as a moderately loud radio, may be identified as aversive if the individual will engage in a behavior such as turning a control knob in order to reduce or terminate the stimulus. Aversive stimuli may be either those events which are physically painful or events which have acquired aversive properties, such as criticism, loss of privileges, or stimuli which signify the approaching occurrence of an aversive event. Just as in the case of a positive reinforcer, events which may be aversive on one occasion may not be on another, and events which may not be aversive to one individual may be highly aversive to another.

Neutral Stimuli. There are a wide variety of stimulus events constantly occurring in a natural environment, such as the honking of a car horn, the ticking of a clock, and the sound of background music, which usually neither increase nor decrease the frequency of a given behavior. Such stimuli may be classified as neutral stimuli. It is important to note, however, that neutral stimuli frequently assume reinforcing properties, either positive or negative, under certain specific conditions discussed below.

Conditioned Reinforcers

The great majority of stimulus events which control complex human behavior are conditioned reinforcers which have no inherent biologic reinforcing value to the organism. Conditioned reinforcers and how to potentiate them assume major significance in behavior control in the dental setting where it is usually impractical, inefficient, or impossible to use a primary reinforcer such as food.

The general procedure for potentiating a neutral stimulus as a conditioned reinforcer is to pair it with a reinforcing stimulus or to arrange conditions so that the neutral stimulus becomes a means toward obtaining a desired reinforcer. For example, money may have little or no reinforcing value for a young child until it becomes a means toward obtaining some desired trinket or toy.

One system of conditioned reinforcement which has proven highly effective in behavior control is the *token reinforcement system*.[7, 10] In this system some tangible stimulus such as a poker chip, a marble, a gold star, or a simple checkmark is designated as the token or the conditioned reinforcer. The system is arranged so that a token is delivered immediately after each occurrence of the desired behavior. After a prespecified number of tokens have been accumulated the child may exchange them for some desired prize reward or privilege. The advantage of this system is that it provides for immediate reinforcement of appropriate behavior and at the same time allows for considerable delay in delivery of the primary reinforcer.

Stimulus Control

The preceding discussion has stressed the importance of consequences in the control of behavior. It is also necessary to account for the fact that a tremendous amount of our behavior appears to be controlled by stimuli which precede the response. We stop our car in the presence of a red light, but not in the presence of a green light; we lift the receiver when the telephone rings, but not when it is silent; we rush to be of assistance in the presence of a cry of distress, but not in the absence of such a cry. The apparent control exerted by antecedent stimuli appears initially to represent an exception to the general principle of behavior control by subsequent stimuli. In actual fact, the antecedent stimuli have no controlling properties in and of themselves. Their ability to control behavior derives entirely from the fact that they are discriminative for either positive reinforcement or aversive consequences. If the consequences are changed, the behavior in response to the antecedent stimulus will also change. Consider, for example, that the controlling properties exerted by the red stop light could easily be reversed by a change in the law making red a signal to move and green a signal to stop. The color of the light itself exerts no physical control over our behavior.

Verbal Instruction as a Form of Stimulus Control

Since so much human behavior is controlled by verbal instruction in the form of requests, commands, or simple communication, it is often assumed that the control exerted by verbal behavior occupies a special status. In the dental office as elsewhere, children are expected to obey, to follow instructions, and to comply with requests. When they do not, the child's failure to comply is often attributed to some internal variable such as negativism or poor motivation, over which it is assumed that the dentist has little control. In actual fact, the control exerted by verbal behavior occupies precisely the same status as the control exerted by other antecedent stimuli discussed above; that is, its controlling properties derive entirely from the consequences attached to the behavior under instructional control. If the positive reinforcement normally associated with following instructions is removed, or if following instructions results in aversive stimuli rather than positive reinforcement, as may be the case in the dental situation, then the control normally exerted by verbal behavior will be lost.

Losing and Regaining Stimulus Control

Understanding that antecedent stimuli derive their controlling properties from the consequences normally associated with them provides the dentist with a much more effective approach to controlling behavior when stimulus or instructional control is lost. If a child who is usually quite cooperative and responsive to verbal directions by the dentist suddenly becomes unmanageable and unresponsive, the most effective approach toward regaining behavior control is to focus upon the identification of powerful positive reinforcers and make them contingent upon the desired behavior. Such a procedure is usually much more effective than attempting to regain control through coaxing, physical restraint, threats, or appeals to what the child should do. Only to the extent that verbal instructions and requests are discriminative for reinforcement will they control behavior.

PRODUCING BEHAVIOR CHANGE

When a program is undertaken in a dental setting, the behavioral goals may be divided into three general categories, namely, (1) new behaviors which one wishes to produce, (2) existing behaviors which one wishes to maintain or strengthen, and (3) existing behaviors which one wishes to eliminate or decrease in frequency. Four basic procedures with which the pedodontist should become familiar are usually used together in producing new complex behaviors.

Procedures for Developing New Behaviors

Shaping

The most effective and most frequently used procedure for producing new behaviors is through a technique termed *shaping*. This is a technique whereby the desired behavior is clearly specified in objective terms and analyzed into its component and sequential parts. As soon as the child engages in any small approximation to the desired terminal behavior he is immediately reinforced. After each response that more closely approximates the desired behavior, he is again reinforced. If, for example, the desired behavior is to have a resistant child sit quietly in the dental chair, the child would first be reinforced for looking in the direction of the chair, then for taking a step in the direction of the chair, then for touching the chair, and finally for sitting in the chair. After the child was seated in the chair he would be reinforced on a periodic basis for remaining seated quietly in the dental chair.

Importance of the Time Relationship between Response and Reinforcement

Since the importance of both reward and punishment in the control of behavior has long been recognized, it may not be readily apparent how current behavior technology differs from previous, more general uses of praise and punishment. The high degree of behavioral control which can be achieved through operant conditioning results primarily from one factor, namely, the precise administration of reinforcement immediately following each small component part of the desired terminal response. It has been demonstrated that a difference in timing of no more than 1 to 2 seconds can alter the form of the behavior which will be reinforced and strengthened.[4] Furthermore, the strengthening of behavior through the administration of reinforcement is not dependent upon the patient's understanding the purpose of reinforcement. Thus the behavior of a patient may be very precisely manipulated without his knowledge as long as reinforcement is administered immediately following the desired response. The degree of skill required to identify precisely the desired behavior and to administer reinforcement at exactly the correct moment is quite similar to the precision skill required in other aspects of dental therapy.

Prompting

If the child makes absolutely no voluntary approximation to the desired behavior, some form of physical prompting may be employed. For example, if the desired behavior is to have the child open his mouth on command, but the child sits with his teeth tightly clenched, a prompting procedure may be used to initiate the desired chain of behavior. In this case the dentist would ask the child to open his mouth and simultaneously touch the child's lip very lightly, depress it slightly, and then praise the child for "opening his mouth," even though the teeth remained clenched. This procedure would continue until the child voluntarily opened his lips on command. The same technique would be used in order to have the child open his mouth completely. The teeth would be parted very slightly and the child would again by praised and rewarded for "opening his mouth." Such a procedure will usually result in acquisition of the desired behavior in a relatively short period of time.

Fading

Fading is a companion procedure whereby control of a behavior is transferred from one stimulus to another and is frequently used in conjunction with the prompting procedure. In the example given above, the initial stimulus controlling the opening of the mouth is the pedodontist's touch on the lip of the child. Since, however, the desired response is that the child will open his mouth at the verbal request of the dentist, the control must be gradually shifted from the tactile stimulus to the verbal stimulus. The verbal stimulus "open your mouth" is, therefore, given simultaneously with the tactile stimulus on the child's lip. Very gradually over a series of several trials the tactile stimulus is "faded" out, leaving only the verbal stimulus in control of the behavior.

Chaining

Chaining is a procedure whereby a series of relatively discrete behaviors which have been individually shaped or conditioned are linked together to form one complex behavioral chain. The dentist may initially shape and reinforce a series of discrete behaviors, such as remaining quiet in the office, climbing into the dental chair, opening the mouth, and keeping the mouth open during the dental procedures. After the separate behaviors have been individually conditioned, they can be incorporated into one smooth behavioral chain by providing reinforcement upon completion of one behavior which leads directly into the next behavior in the sequence. For example, as soon as the child sits quietly in the dental chair, the dentist might say, "That's excellent, I'm so proud of you for sitting in the chair that I'm going to give you a gold star, *and as soon as you open your mouth I have another one for you.*" Similar "double" reinforcement instructions are provided at the end of each behavior so that each step blends smoothly and naturally into the next.

Procedures for Increasing or Maintaining the Strength of Existing Behaviors

After a new behavior has been shaped or conditioned, one of the most effective methods for maintaining or increasing the strength of the response is through the procedure of *intermittent reinforcement.* In contrast to the procedure for shaping a new behavior which requires administration of reinforcement following each response, intermittent reinforcement is a procedure whereby reinforcement is administered only after a specific number of responses or after a specific amount of time has elapsed. When a specific number of responses are required for reinforcement, the schedule is termed a *ratio schedule,* and when a set amount of time must elapse prior to reinforcement the schedule is termed an *interval schedule.* The most familiar example of intermittent reinforcement is the slot machine gambling device which rewards or reinforces only after a specific but unpredictable number of responses have occurred. Such a schedule of reinforcement, termed a *variable ratio schedule,* is capable of maintaining a tremendously high response rate over an extended period of time with a minimum of reinforcement. Translated into the dental setting this means that after the pedodontist has successfully conditioned good dental behavior in his patients, such behavior may be maintained relatively easily over a long period of time by providing praise or other conditioned reinforcement on a very intermittent schedule.

Procedures for Decreasing the Frequency of a Behavior through the Use of Positive Reinforcement

A major area of concern with children who are considered behavior problems in the dental setting is usually the elimination of some undesirable behavior such as hitting, screaming, or crying. A number of effective techniques for reducing problem behavior which rely primarily upon manipulation of positive reinforcement have been developed.

Extinction

Since behavior is maintained by reinforcement, the elimination of reinforcement will result in the gradual elimination or extinction of the behavior. Experimentally this procedure is one of the easiest to implement because it involves only the identification and elimination of reinforcement. From a practical standpoint, however, the procedure may not be the technique of choice in the dental setting because the method is relatively slow, because it is frequently impossible to identify the reinforcer, and because it is often impossible to eliminate the reinforcer even if it can be identified.

Time Out

Time out is a modification of the extinction procedure which involves removing the child briefly from a reinforcing situation contingent upon an undesired response. Thus if a child should begin to cry during the treatment process, the dentist could withdraw social reinforcement by turning away from the child for a few seconds.

Response Cost

Response cost is procedurally similar to time out, but in this case some tangible reinforcer is actually taken from the child contingent upon the undesired response. For example, if the child has earned a large number of points or tokens for good dental behavior, a certain number of tokens would be lost when the child engaged in an inappropriate behavior.

Reinforcement of an Incompatible Response

Probably the most effective clinical technique for rapidly eliminating an undesirable response is to reinforce the child for engaging in a behavior which is incompatible with the undesirable response while simultaneously removing reinforcement from the undesired behavior. For example, if elimination of crying is the desired behavioral goal, the child would receive no reinforcement in the form of attention or other rewards while crying but would be rewarded instantly upon termination of crying. Reinforcement would then continue on an intermittent schedule as long as the child remained silent, a response which is, of course, incompatible with crying.

Using Aversive Control Techniques

While the preferred method of behavior control is through the use of positive reinforcement, it is also true that aversive techniques can be used both to increase the frequency of a desired response and to decrease the frequency of an undesired response. It is therefore important to understand the procedures and to recognize some of the disadvantages inherent in the use of aversive techniques.

Punishment-Decreasing Response Frequency

When aversive stimuli are used to decrease the frequency of a behavior, the technique is termed *punishment*. Punishment involves the administration of an aversive stimulus immediately after the undesired behavior occurs. The aversive stimulus may be a painful physical stimulus, such as a slap or a loud, high pitched tone, or it may be a conditioned aversive stimulus such as a sharp, "No!" In general, one may expect punishment procedures to produce a decrease in the frequency of the undesired behavior. Frequently, however, paradoxical results are obtained, and an increase rather than a decrease in the frequency of the behavior will occur. For this reason, the use of punishment procedures in the dental situation is not normally recommended.

Negative Reinforcement—Increasing a Desired Behavior

While use of aversive stimuli to decrease an undesired behavior in a punishment paradigm is a relatively familiar procedure, it is not so well known that aversive techniques can be used to increase the rate of a desired behavior. If contingencies are arranged so that the occurrence of the desired behavior will eliminate an aversive stimulus, the behavior which eliminates the stimulus will increase in frequency. In *negative reinforcement* two basic procedures may be used, namely, an *escape procedure* and an *avoidance procedure*. In the escape procedure the aversive stimulus is actually administered, and the subject must engage in a specified response to eliminate or escape from the aversive stimulus. For example, the dentist might physically restrain a screaming child and release him only after a brief period of silence.

In the avoidance paradigm, the subject may avoid the aversive stimulus altogether by engaging in the appropriate response prior to administration of the aversive stimulus. Thus the dentist might say to a child, "Unless you sit quietly in the chair, we will have to restrain your arms and legs." If the child becomes quiet, he successfully avoids restraint.

Disadvantages of Aversive Control

While the aversive control procedures can in some cases be effective agents of behavior control, there are a number of reasons why aversive techniques are not generally recommended in behavior control work, and why they should be used sparingly and with judicious restraint in the dental setting.

Risk of Trauma to the Child.   A large number of aversive techniques contain within them the risk of possible injury to the child, if not directly from the procedure itself, then from the child's attempts to escape from the situation. The dentist may, of course, be held legally responsible for any adverse effects the child might suffer.

Disrupting Desirable Behavior Patterns.   Aversive stimuli frequently produce emotional responses which can totally disrupt, in a short time, desirable behavioral patterns which may have taken months or years to condition. At the very least, there is a risk of decreasing the frequency of many of the very behaviors which the dentist wishes to build up.

Creating Fears, Phobias, and Other Avoidance Behaviors.   The short-term gains achieved through the use of aversive techniques to suppress temper tantrums and other similar behaviors may be completely outweighed by creation of a deeply entrenched dental phobia which may result in future avoidance of the entire dental situation.   The case discussed later in this paper is an example of a dental phobia created through the use of aversive techniques.

Producing Aggressive Behavior.   Aversive techniques frequently create aggressive and attack behavior directed against the agent of aversive control. Thus, if aversive techniques are used to control a child, the child, if he is physically able, is quite apt to direct physical aggression toward the dentist who uses aversive techniques. At the very least, the child may be quite hostile toward the dentist.

Aversive Techniques Are Reinforcing to the User.   Because aversive control techniques frequently do produce rather rapid short-term results, particularly in the suppression of behavior, dentists who use such procedures can easily fall into the trap of relying increasingly upon aversive controls until they find themselves in highly embarrassing legal or professional situations. Such cases are already a matter of record in behavior therapy. Because of these and other undesirable side effects, it is recommended that positive reinforcement procedures be relied upon as the primary method of choice and supplemented only on rare occasions by the use of aversive control.

IMPLEMENTING A BEHAVIOR MODIFICATION PROGRAM
IN THE DENTAL SETTING

The dental setting is in many ways ideally suited to the use of behavioral techniques. All of the desired behavior takes place in the limited confines of the dental office, and the target behavior, that of cooperation, is similar for all patients and can easily be analyzed into its component parts for shaping. Moreover, the dentist has at his immediate disposal a variety of reinforcers which can be used.

Basic Steps in Implementing a Program

To design an effective behavior modification program, certain basic information is required in almost every case.

Identification of the desired target behavior or terminal response repertoire

In the dental setting, the overall behavior goal will usually be the same for most children, that is, to have the child walk quietly and voluntarily into the dental office, get into the treatment chair, and sit quietly and cooperatively during treatment.

Identification of specific behaviors to be produced or conditioned

Using the desired terminal behavioral repertoire as a guide, the initial behavior of the child is evaluated in order to determine what new behaviors must be produced. For example, a child may be generally pleasant and cooperative, but may totally refuse to get into the treatment chair. This then becomes the immediate target behavior to be shaped.

Identification of undesirable behaviors to be weakened or eliminated

Many children who are considered behavior management problems exhibit a relatively large number of undesirable behaviors. While many of these behaviors, such as screaming, may be incompatible with the acquisition of good dental behavior, others, such as a generally negative attitude, may not be. The task of the dentist is to identify in precise operational terms those behaviors which he must decrease in frequency before dental work can proceed.

Determination of effective reinforcers

Since the success of a behavior modification program rests heavily upon the availability of appropriate reinforcing stimuli, it is essential to identify at the outset those reinforcers which will control the behavior of the child.

This can be accomplished relatively quickly and efficiently through the procedure termed *reinforcement sampling*. The child is given an opportunity to look at, hold, taste, or listen to a variety of potential reinforcers which the dentist has available in his office. Such a display is termed a *reinforcement menu*. Those items in which the child displays high interest will in most cases serve as reinforcers.

Determination of procedures for recording, timing, and tabulation of data

Although formal tabulation of behavioral data may not be necessary in all cases, behavior modification programs are based upon the premise that the reinforcement procedures used will, in fact, produce a measurable change in the frequency of the target behavior. An effective data recording system will give immediate feedback regarding effectiveness of the program. If no measurable change in the target behavior occurs, the procedures must be modified. While major changes in behavior, such as a rapid and dramatic decrease in rate of crying, can be observed without benefit of measuring devices, other changes in behavior, such as a slight increase in the length of time that a child keeps his mouth open, may be impossible to assess without benefit of mechanical recording devices. It is, therefore, desirable to have available, as minimum equipment, a stopwatch, a counter, and a data sheet on which to record behavior frequency on a time base. A particularly useful five-channel, manually operated mechanical counter (Multi-Counter #99C9031) can be obtained from Lafayette Radio and Electronics, 111 Jericho Turnpike, Syosset, L.I., New York, 11791. More elaborate recording equipment can be obtained from Tech Ser, Inc., 5301 Holland Drive, Beltsville, Maryland, 20705.

Outlining the reinforcement program or the shaping sequence

After the basic details of identifying target behaviors, reinforcers, and recording procedures have been completed, the next step is to outline, either formally or informally, a tentative sequential program for moving the child from the baseline performance level to the desired target behavior. This is the heart of the behavior modification program and must be individually tailored to the behavior of each child. This usually involves an identification of the various behaviors required to reach the final target performance and a sequencing of the behaviors in a logical step-by-step fashion so that at each stage of the reinforcement program, the child has mastered all of the previous steps. The initial program serves as a guide to action, but it should be considered tentative in the sense that, if during programming it becomes obvious that the sequence should be changed or that additional behaviors are needed, appropriate revisions are made in the program.

An Illustrative Case Study

Background

Debbie R. was a 12-year-old white female of normal intelligence who was referred because she was a severe management problem. She had been treated previously in a private dental setting, and all dental treatment had to be administered under general anesthesia. Prior to referral, the child had refused to keep any further dental appointments and had begun to develop a generalized fear of all medical and dental settings. She was referred to the Kennedy Institute where a behavior modification program was to be implemented in conjunction with the dental treatment.

Session 1 (10-20-72)

The first session was used primarily as a baseline to determine the severity of the child's behavior problem, to determine what reinforcers might be effective and to explain the reforcement program to the child and her parents. The child was extremely reluctant to approach the treatment room, but did so with forceful urging from her parents. As soon as the child entered the treatment room, she was immediately put at ease by praising her for coming into the treatment room and complimenting her on her appearance. Since she was obviously quite responsive to social reinforcement, this was continued and the child was also assured that she would be able to participate in a new type of dental game in which she could win various prizes for good behavior. With this assurance plus a high degree of social reinforcement, the child allowed her parents to leave the treatment room.

After further discussion of the reward game, the child agreed to allow the dentist to take x-rays, on the condition that absolutely no treatment would be performed on her teeth. The child was lavishly praised both during the x-ray procedure and immediately thereafter. She was also told that she had accumulated enough points to win a prize from the reinforcement menu which consisted of happy-face stickers, tooth paste, toothbrushes, mouthwash, and a variety of small toys. By the end of the session the child was smiling, happy, and obviously pleased with herself. She was relaxed enough to discuss her doubts and fears regarding dental treatment and revealed the significant fact that her fears stemmed primarily from being slapped by a dentist during treatment when she was a young child. She readily agreed to return for a second session during which she could win additional prizes and during which it was mutually agreed that the only treatment to be performed would be a dental prophylaxis.

Session 2 (10-27-72)

During the second session a full-mouth scaling and polishing were performed. A high density of praise and social reinforcement was administered throughout treatment, contingent upon cooperative dental behavior. The patient, though initially apprehensive, came under rapid control by the positive social reinforcement and was cooperative during the entire treatment session. At the end of the session, the child was again praised for her excellent dental behavior, was told that she had won enough points for two prizes and was again given her choice of treats from the reinforcement menu. The child readily agreed to a third appointment. By the end of this session, it was apparent that social reinforcement and praise were beginning to assume major control over the child's behavior and were at least as effective in behavior control as were the tangible rewards which were of negligible monetary value.

Session 3 (12-4-72)

The patient was initially quite apprehensive since she was aware that dental repair work was to be done. As soon as the patient arrived, however, all three staff members, the dentist, the psychologist, and the dental hygienist administered continuous positive reinforcement for even the most inconsequential cooperative behaviors and continually reminded her that she was rapidly accumulating large numbers of points toward a very special prize which we had for her at the end of the session. The procedure was highly successful in that the only negative reaction of the child during the entire session was a few tears during administration of a local anesthetic. One tooth was treated and the session was intentionally kept very short. As soon as the session was over, the child was lavishly praised for her excellent behavior, allowed to choose a prize from the reinforcement menu, and then as a special surprise reward, she was given a 20-ounce size bottle of mouthwash. The patient was obviously thrilled with the special reward and readily agreed to another treatment session.

Session 4 (12-11-72)

In order to analyze the interaction between the dentist and patient, a tabulation was made of the dentist's behavior and the patient's behavior during each of the 23 1-minute intervals of the treatment session. The dentist had by this time become quite proficient at providing positive reinforcement throughout the session. The data indicated that the dentist provided reinforcing comments or conversation during each of the 1-minute intervals of the session. In addition, the dentist specifically awarded points on nine different occasions, each time following an appropriate behavior such as cooperation during administration of a local anesthetic. The child's response was very positive. She engaged in conversation with the dentist throughout the session, and she smiled or laughed during 13 of the 23 1-minute intervals. Two separate fillings were completed during this session, and there were no instances of negative behavior. The child again received a reward at the end of the session.

Session 5 (12-18-72)

The patient came in to review oral hygiene techniques. She was very positive toward the entire staff and brought in Christmas presents for everyone. This, of course, represented a complete reversal of her initial fearful, resistant attitude.

Session 6 (1-17-73)

The dentist's behavior and the patient's behavior were also tabulated during each of the 26 1-minute intervals of Session 6. The dentist again conducted dental therapy and provided general reinforcing comments during each of the 26 1-minute intervals. In addition he commented "very good" 15 times, contingent on specific cooperative behavior, such as leaning back in the chair and opening the mouth. The patient accumulated a total of 15 points for good behavior during the session and received a reward. No uncooperative or negative behavior occurred.

Session 7 (1-24-73)

This final session was conducted by the dentist without the psychologist present to determine if there would be any change in the patient's behavior. Dental repair work was conducted and the dentist continued the positive reinforcement procedures. The patient's behavior was as positive and as cooperative as on all other occasions and a reward was given at the end of the session. Following this session the mother called to express her appreciation for the complete reversal in the child's attitude toward dental work.

Epilogue

Several months after the final session, the patient and her mother were involved in an accidental explosion in the home which produced burns over 80 per cent of the child's body. Because of the child's previous phobic reaction toward all medical settings, the mother feared the child might become hysterical during hospitalization. In actual fact, the child was a model patient, joked with the staff, and was completely cooperative during treatment. Following her release from the hospital, the mother called to thank the dental staff for the tremendous change which had been produced in the child's attitude toward medical and dental treatment as a result of the positive reinforcement methods.

Discussion

The present case illustrates a number of points regarding the use of behavior modification procedures in the dental setting. First and most significant is the fact that a longstanding history of fear of dental treatment was completely reversed in the course of seven relatively short sessions during which positive reinforcement procedures were used. Second, the case incidentally demonstrates the detrimental effects which can occur through the use of aversive techniques. The child was apparently traumatized on only one occasion several years previously and had feared dental treatment since that time.

Another point of importance to those considering the practical aspects of implementing a behavioral program is that the behavior modification procedures used in this case were essentially quite simple and very easy to implement. The basic steps were, (a) putting the child totally at ease during the first session through extensive use of positive social reinforcement, (b) explaining to the child a very simple reward system, (c) providing constant positive social reinforcement throughout each session, (d) providing verbal praise immediately and very precisely following each bit of desired behavior, (e) providing points verbally each time a desired behavior occurred, (f) ensuring that the points the child earned always entitled her to a prize at the end of the session, (g) avoiding discussion of any negative aspects of dental work during treatment, (h) in addition to awarding the prize, each session was always ended with lavish praise for the child's good behavior.

Finally, it is important to observe that the dentist, who had no previous training in behavior modification, was able to use the procedures quite effectively by the fourth session. After the third session, the psychologist assumed the role of an observer and was primarily responsible for providing a post-session analysis of the treatment procedures.

SUMMARY

Behavior management problems occur frequently in the practice of pediatric dentistry and are especially common in pediatric dental work with the mentally retarded or the emotionally disturbed child. In the past the pedodontist has had few options in dealing with behavior problems other than physical restraint, sedation, or general anesthesia. There are now available to the pedodontist a variety of highly specific behavior modification techniques which will allow the dentist to increase vastly the degree to which he can successfully manage children with behavior problems. The present article summarizes the basic reinforcement techniques which can be used by the pedodontist and presents an illustrative case in which a longstanding dental phobia was reversed in only seven sessions through the use of positive reinforcement.

REFERENCES

1. Baily, P. M., Talbot, A., and Taylor, P. P.: A comparison of maternal anxiety levels with anxiety levels manifested in the child dental patient. *J. Dent. Child., 40*:278, 1973.
2. Blackham, G. J., and Silberman, A.: *Modification of Child Behavior.* Belmont, Calif., Wadsworth Publishing Co., 1971.
3. Drash, P. W., and Freeman, B. J.: *Behavior Modification, Behavior Therapy, and Operant Conditioning: An Historical Survey* and a *Bibliography of Books in Print, 1900-1972.* Baltimore, Behavior Information and Technology, 1973.
4. Ferster, C. B., and Perrott, M. C.: *Behavior Principles.* New York: Appleton-Century-Crofts, 1968.
5. Jenks, L.: How the dentist's behavior can influence the child's behavior. *J. Dent. Child., 31*:358, 1964.
6. Johnson, R., and Machen, J. B.: Behavior modification techniques and maternal anxiety. *J. Dent. Child., 40*:272, 1973.
7. Kazdin, A. E., and Bootzin, R. R.: The token economy: an evaluative review. *J. Applied Behav. Anal., 5*:343, 1972.
8. Kleinknecht, R. A., Klepac, R. K., and Alexander, L. D.: Origins and characteristics of fear of dentistry. *J.A.D.A., 86*:842, 1973.
9. Kohlenberg, R., Greenberg, D., Reymore, L., and Hass, G.: Behavior modification and the management of mentally retarded dental patients. *J. Dent. Child., 39*:61, 1972.
10. Sulzer, B., and Mayer, G. R.: *Behavior Modification Procedures for School Personnel.* Hinsdale, Ill., Dryden Press, 1972.
11. Wright, G. Z., Alpern, G. D., and Leake, J. L.: The modifiability of maternal anxiety as it relates to children's cooperative dental behavior. *J. Dent. Child., 40*:265, 1973.

4

VISION

INTRODUCTION

Though vision is one of the most important of the senses, little has been done in either the behavioral analysis of vision and its maladies or the study of the use of various behavioral techniques in the treatment of visual dysfunction. Brady and Lind (1961) were among the first to perform an experimental analysis of hysterical blindness. They utilized operant techniques to demonstrate that the behavior of an adult patient who claimed to be blind could be controlled by visual stimuli. In a follow-up to that study, Grosz and Zimmerman (1970) showed that the clinical improvement obtained in the hospital did not maintain when the patient was released from the hospital.

In an article by Ohno and associates (Ohno, Sugita, Takeya, Akagi, Tanaka & Ikemi, 1974), three cases of hysterical blindness in adults and the application of behavioral techniques were described. Stolz and Wolf (1969) presented an experimental analysis of a 16-year-old retarded male who was diagnosed as organically blind. Their results showed that, given practice in discriminating visual stimuli, self-help skills were enhanced. Similarly, Grosz and Zimmerman (1970) described the application of behavioral techniques to a functionally blind adolescent girl.

Other studies with adults have involved attempts at modification of refractory error through conditioning (Giddings & Lanyon, 1974), the treatment of a chronic eye closure reaction (Norton 1976), and the treatment of tic-like high rate blinking, or blepharospasm (Sharpe, 1974). Goldblatt and Steisel (1973) discussed the applications of behavioral techniques with multiply handicapped blind children. In a similar article, Craig and Holland (1970) explored the reinforcement of visual attending in classrooms for deaf children. Unlike the children's dentist, the vision specialist generally provides relatively innocuous methods for adherence to a treatment regimen. With perhaps the exception of the use of eyedrops to dilate the eyes and related procedures for ophthalmological examinations, the visit to the ophthalmologist becomes an interesting experience for the young child. The ophthalmologist or optometrist can generally complete a clinical exam and prescribe the prosthesis without difficulty, but then runs into a substantial problem of ensuring compliance with the treatment prescribed, such as wearing glasses. The vision specialist must frequently depend on the parent or the teacher to assure sufficient compliance with the prescribed treatment in order to allow adequate corrective measures.

Wolf, Risley, and Mees (1964) summarized their work with a three-year-old childhood schizophrenic. At the age of nine months, "Dicky" was discovered to have severe cataracts on both eyes and was beginning to develop temper tantrums and sleeping problems. Upon Dicky's admission to the hospital, the ophthalmologist diagnosed him as needing glasses, without which he would lose his macular vision in six weeks. The authors present detailed treatment procedures, using shaping, for getting him to accept the wearing of glasses, starting with the presentation of empty rings and, though a series of approximations, to wearing the complete glass frame. After accepting glasses Dicky developed the behavior of throwing them; but with the use of time-out following each incident of glasses throwing, the behavior was quickly eliminated. The authors also illustrate the application of their techniques to other associated disruptive behavior, such as sleeping, eating, and talking. Developmentally handicapped children like Dicky present an interesting challenge to behavior therapists in that they seldom treat one or two isolated behaviors but must contend with a number of them.

Visual training has long been used by optometrists to treat strabismus, limitation of gaze, excess or insufficient conversions, and ptosis. Letourneau (1976) and Letourneau and Ludlam (1976), for example, describe their work with children using behavior modification and biofeedback to assist in visual retraining. Included in this chapter is an article by Ulan, Juris, and Dornback (1974) in which they present techniques used in the treatment of an amblyopic child. Behavioral techniques were used to get the child to accept the wearing of an eye patch sufficiently long to provide adequate correction. They describe the use of successive approximation to shape the child's patch-wearing behavior from 15 minutes to an optimal period, and illustrate step-by-step techniques that can be used to teach parents how to keep patches on their difficult children. These simple techniques can be easily taught to most parents in the vision specialist's office.

References

Brady, J. P., & Lind, D. L. Experimental analysis of hysterical blindness. *Archives of General Psychiatry*, 1961, *4*, 331-339.

Craig, H. B., & Holland, A. L. Reinforcement of visual attending in classrooms of deaf children. *Journal of Applied Behavior Analysis*, 1970, *3*, 97-109.

Giddings, J. W., & Lanyon, R. I. Modification of refractory error through conditioning: An exploratory study. *Behavior Therapy*, 1974, *2*, 538-542.

Goldblatt, M., & Steisel, I. M. Behavior modification with multi-handicapped blind children. A paper presented to the American Psychological Association Convention, Montreal, August 29, 1973.

Grosz, H. J., & Zimmerman, J. A second detailed case study of functional blindness: Further demonstration of the contribution of objective psychological laboratory data. *Behavior Therapy*, 1970, *1*, 115-123.

Letourneau, J. E. Application of biofeedback and behavior modification techniques in visual training. *Journal of Optometry and Physiological Optics*, 1976, *53*, 187-190.

Letourneau, J. E., & Ludlam, W. M. Biofeedback reinforcement in the training of limitation of gaze: A case report. *Journal of Optometry and Physiological Optics,* 1976, *53*, 672-676.

Norton, G. R. Biofeedback treatment of long-standing eye closure reactions. *Journal of Behavior Therapy and Experimental Psychiatry*, 1976, *7*, 279-280.

Ohno, Y., Sugita, M., Takeya, T., Akagi, M., Tanaka, Y., & Ikemi, Y. The treatment of hysterical blindness by behavioral therapy. *Psychosomatics,* 1974, *15*, 79-82.

Sharpe, R. Behavior therapy in a case of blepharospasm. *British Journal of Psychiatry*, 1974, *124*, 603-604.

Stolz, S. B., & Wolf, M. M. Visually discriminated behavior in a "blind" adolescent retardate. *Journal of Applied Behavior Analysis*, 1969, *2*, 65-77.

Ulan, H., Juris, A., & Dornback, F. Keeping that patch on: The application of behavioral modification techniques in orthoptic practice. *American Orthoptic Journal*, 1974, *24*, 60-62.

Wolf, M., Risley, T., & Mees, H. Application of operant conditioning procedures to the behavior problems of an autistic child. *Behaviour Research and Therapy*, 1964, *1*, 305-312.

KEEPING THAT PATCH ON:
THE APPLICATION
OF BEHAVIOR MODIFICATION TECHNIQUES
IN ORTHOPTIC PRACTICE

Howard Ulan
Antoinette Juris
Fred Dornback

A problem frequently encountered in orthoptic practice is the tendency of some young amblyopic patients to resist the wearing of an eye patch. Parents of such a patient may report that the child sometimes removes the patch after wearing it only a few minutes, or in some cases, after about an hour. Obviously, therapeutic progress is greatly hindered by this kind of behavior. Many parents attempt to cope with this problem by punishing the child for removing the patch. This method often fails, however, and it may have undesirable side effects, such as arousing anger and resentment in the child.

A more effective way of dealing with problems of this sort is to apply the reinforcement techniques pioneered by Skinner.[1] These methods have been widely used in recent years in the correction of maladaptive behavior of many kinds.[2-4] According to these principles, the frequency of virtually any type of behavior can be increased by following the specified behavior with a reinforcing event. We say that a response is positively reinforced when a positive reinforcer is presented following the response. Generally, a positive reinforcer is a reward. Positive reinforcers may be tangible things, such as candy or toys, or privileges, such as going to a park or to a movie, or attention or signs of approval from others. It is important to realize that what is reinforcing for one person may not be reinforcing for another and something which is reinforcing at one time

Reprinted from the *American Orthoptic Journal*, 1974, *24*, 60-62. Copyright 1974 by the American Academy of Opthalmology and Otolaryngology. Reprinted by permission.

Howard Ulan is at Alma College, Alma, Michigan. Antoinette Juris is in the Ophthalmology Department of Evanston Hospital in Evanston, Illinois. Fred Dornback is in the North Suburban Special Education District in Highland Park, Illinois.

may not be so at another time. A little experimentation may be necessary to determine what is most effective for a given individual.

An important aspect of the reinforcement procedure is the technique of behavior shaping through the use of successive approximations. If the desired behavior is not currently being emitted by the patient, we cannot reasonably wait for it to occur in order to reinforce it. Instead, we should reinforce any behavior which is similar to or which contributes in some way to the desired behavior, and then gradually shift the criterion for reinforcement closer and closer to this behavior. Suppose that we want a child to wear an eye patch all day, but the child removes it after wearing it about 15 minutes. Initially, we would reinforce the child's behavior any time he left it on for longer than 15 minutes, then only after 30 minutes, then after an hour, and so on. The precise time intervals are not important, but the principle of gradually making them longer is.

In order to know what duration of patch-wearing behavior should initially be required before the reinforcer is presented, the parent may keep a record of the average amount of time the child wears the patch before removing it. If, prior to the initiation of the behavior modification program, the child wears the patch an average of 30 minutes before removing it, the reinforcer should be presented each time he wears the patch for 30 minutes or longer, but not if he removes the patch after wearing it less than 30 minutes. After having been reinforced for wearing the patch for 30 minutes or longer periods, the child should be keeping the patch on for longer periods more frequently. When this occurs, still longer periods of patch-wearing behavior should be required before reinforcement is provided. While this behavior-shaping procedure is being used it is important that the parents not make a big fuss whenever the child removes the patch before the criterion is met, since attention of this sort may itself be reinforcing, and the parent would be reinforcing the *undesirable* behavior of removing the patch.

Instead, the parent should replace the eye patch in a perfunctory manner whenever it is removed prematurely, and briefly explain to the child that if the patch is worn for the specified period of time, the reinforcer will be provided.

One of us (A.J.) has recommended these techniques to ten mothers who had difficulty keeping a patch on their children. The method was described to the mother and she was given the following written instructions:

MAKING IT WORTHWHILE TO WEAR AN EYE PATCH

"Your child is going to have to wear a patch on his or her eye. Because this is frequently more important to us as adults than it is to the child, it becomes necessary to work with the child on this project.

"The following are some simple but significant points that may benefit your child and allow you to be more comfortable in dealing with him/her during this period of therapy.

"Our program is frequently called 'Behavior Modification.' Let me define my terms.

A. Behavior—behavior is anything that we can see or hear. In other words, 'anyone' could tell it was happening or not happening. Wearing an eye patch is a behavior. Writing, talking, and standing are also behavior.

B. Modification—this means we will change something. An example is that your child previously did not wear a patch and now he must. This is modification.

"A second area of importance is this 'Behavior' is learned by reinforcement. By this we mean we do things because we see them as worthwhile. We may see it as worthwhile because we think it important OR because someone trying to modify our behavior is trying to help us learn that the behavior is worthwhile doing. You may try several ways, such as *social reinforcement*—praise, hugs, hand shakes, smiles, etc.—or *material reinforcement*. Material reinforcement may include candy, trinkets, toys, or any special privilege.

"A key point is this: 'CATCH THEM BEING GOOD.' The heart of the program says to us that we must give of ourselves in order to influence behavior in others. Translated this means you want your child to learn to wear his eye patch. In an attempt to accomplish this you will try to 'catch the child being good' (WEARING EYE PATCH), and acknowledge it in a way important to the child. If you catch the child being good in a way meaningful to the child, the chances of the child trying to wear the patch or continuing to wear the patch are improved.

"If this doesn't improve the amount of time the child actually wears the patch, one of the things that's wrong may be:

A. What you are offering as reinforcement may not be important enough to the child.

B. You may not be catching the child being good often enough. Remember, 'little steps for little feet.'

"Little steps for little feet means to us that if your child only wears the patch for about two hours, anything above that time would be improvement. If we can improve the eye patch behavior to an average of 2½ hours, we have made a little step toward our goal of full time patch wearing. After 2½ hours occurs with some regularity, we then take another step and another."

Follow-up data are available in eight of the ten cases in which this instruction in behavior modification techniques was provided. These cases included boys and girls, ages 4 to 10 years. In six of the eight cases, the mothers reported good results, with the child wearing the patch all day in most of these cases. In some of the cases, application of these procedures for about a week was sufficient to increase eye-patch wearing behavior to a satisfactory extent, and continued use of the extrinsic positive reinforcers became unnecessary. (This commonly occurs in behavior modification; extrinsic reinforcers are helpful in shaping the desired behavior, but may be unnecessary to maintain it.) In some of the cases, however, it seemed necessary or desirable to continue the reinforcement procedures for several months.

The principal problem encountered in the use of this method is in instructing the parents to use it and convincing them that when properly applied, the reinforcement technique will usually be successful. As far as could be ascertained through questioning of the parents, the failures reported earlier resulted from the parents' not following instructions.

In order to increase the probability that the parents will conscientiously follow the instructions, and in order to deal with any other problems that may arise in carrying out the behavior modification program, the orthoptist may be able to enlist the help of the local school psychologist. Some school psychologists are highly skilled in the use of the behavior modification techniques described here, but some are not, and the orthoptist should determine whether the psychologist has this competence. If he does, he can be an important source of help in instructing the patient's parents, and he can also see that these techniques are used by the patient's teachers in school.

In summary, the behavior modification methods described here provide the orthoptist with means to deal with a problem that often arises in treating young amblyopic patients. The simple therapeutic procedure of wearing an eye patch can be of very great benefit, and the orthoptist should take advantage of behavior modification techniques to help ensure that the patch is worn.

REFERENCES

1. Skinner BF: *Science and Human Behavior.* New York: Macmillan Co., 1953.
2. MacMillan D: *Behavior Modification in Education.* New York: Macmillan Co., 1973.
3. Patterson GR, Gullion ME: *Living with Children*, ed 2. Champaign, Ill.: Research Press, 1971.
4. Ullmann LP, Krasner L: *Case Studies in Behavior Modification.* New York: Holt, Rinehart & Winston, 1965.

5

HEARING

INTRODUCTION

Emotionally disturbed deaf children needing audiological evaluation are frequently too disruptive to be tested. Only recently has the training of audiologists and speech and hearing specialists included such techniques as shaping, stimulus control, and token reinforcement. In the past, such children were either untestable or, at best, inadequately tested. In some cases, the psychologically sophisticated hearing expert sought consultation with a behavioral psychologist who may have demonstrated the use of shaping and successive approximation to achieve the desired goal. Speech and hearing personnel now widely utilize shaping procedures, not only for the development of cooperative behaviors to facilitate an optimal hearing evaluation in disturbed children, but even more widely for the treatment of normal deaf children. Behavioral techniques can be used in the therapeutic setting to increase adherence to visual signals, sitting on command, and attending to the task at hand. These techniques, combined with the use of time-out or response-cost and, if necessary, physical punishment, can effectively eliminate distractors and other self-stimulating behaviors.

Once deaf children are evaluated and minimal cooperation elicited, they must be trained to accept and use their expensive, sometimes fragile hearing aids. They must be trained to wear the aids long enough each day to provide the minimum speech and language stimulation to begin language education. They also must be trained not to throw their hearing aids, dunk them in the commode, or do any of the other destructive things that young children think up.

Many hearing disordered children are detected at two to three years of age, the period of drastically accelerated language development, great intellectual curiosity, and increasing individuation and separation from mother. The therapist must influence children to accept their hearing aids, regard them not as toys or objects of experimentation, and exercise compliance beyond that typical of their peers. To achieve these ends, parents must be involved in the development of home programs to maximize hearing skills.

Speech and hearing specialists have long been pioneers in the development of parent education programs to aid the social skills development of these children. Once compliant behavior is obtained in school and clinic, these skills must generalize to the home. With the increased striving for independence of the deaf child, which is usually concurrent with the diagnosis and beginning of treatment, parents need special skills and guidance to deal effectively with this critical developmental phase. Parents of children who are deaf frequently have not accepted their children's limitations and consequently may overprotect them. Disappointment with their less-than-normal children may elicit parental behaviors that frustrate their children and serve to antagonize parent-child relationships, further complicating the educational task of the hearing therapist. Parents, even those supportive and understanding, must be trained to respond effectively to the needs of the children.

Mira (1972) describes a home training program implemented by parents. The procedures outlined capitalize on the close, natural relationship between parents, especially mothers, and their young children. The article deals with problems of inadequacy of verbal controls, childhood negativism, adjustment to prosthetic devices and parents' reactions to the diagnosis of hearing impairment, and offers a practical model for working with children and their families.

In this chapter Garrard and Saxon (1973) describe the steps necessary to prepare a disturbed three-year-old girl for a hearing therapy program. They review a step-by-step procedure for dealing with screaming and crying by shaping of attending behavior, establishing sitting behavior, increasing sitting time, and, finally, modification of screaming behavior. This article emphasizes the importance of preparing children who are deaf or hard-of-hearing for subsequent training by eliminating high rate, disruptive behaviors that interfere with learning.

References

Garrard, K. R., & Saxon, S. A. Preparation of a disturbed deaf child for therapy: A case description in behavior shaping. *Journal of Speech and Hearing Disorders*, 1973, *38*, 502-509.

Mira, M. Behavioral modification applied to training young deaf children. *Exceptional Children*, 1972, *39*, 225-229.

PREPARATION OF A DISTURBED
DEAF CHILD FOR THERAPY:
A CASE DESCRIPTION
IN BEHAVIOR SHAPING

Kay R. Garrard
Samuel A. Saxon

This case report includes a description of a disturbed three-year-old deaf female and the treatment plan followed to prepare for her a hearing therapy program. Particular emphasis is given to the initial steps taken to train the speech pathologist and the patient's mother in behavior modification. Graphs illustrating the patient's progress are presented and described.

The need for programs for multiply handicapped deaf children has been stressed in previous articles by Ladson (1965), Warren (1961), and Withrow (1966). Realizing that traditional methods often do not work with multiply handicapped deaf youngsters, some educators have learned that behavior modification techniques can be powerful tools for modifying and maintaining behaviors necessary for these children to learn. However, as Lennan (1970) pointed out, many who work with the deaf do not use the techniques because of little or no exposure to behavioral technology. Lennan effectively used behavior techniques in a program for emotionally disturbed deaf boys. Salzinger (1970) also supported the use of behavior theory in working with the deaf and suggested that anyone in contact with the deaf learn behavior principles. He defined behavior theory as a system of related principles which allows us to describe, analyze, and control behavior. The use of behavior theory with other populations

Reprinted from *Journal of Speech and Hearing Disorders*, 1978, *38*, 502-509. Copyright 1973 by the American Speech, Language and Hearing Society. Reprinted by permission.

Kay R. Garrard is a Ph.D. candidate in educational psychology, University of California, Berkeley, California. Samuel A. Saxon is at the University of Alabama, Birmingham, Alabama.

suggests that it should aid us in identifying some of the variables that influence the behavior of the deaf and in treating the adjustment problems of the deaf.

Some of the main principles of behavior theory are these: (1) Behavior has consequences; that is, something happens after a response is made. (2) The consequence of a behavior determines whether that behavior will reappear, be it simple or complex, adaptive or maladaptive. (3) A child will perform to obtain a reinforcer, either consumable or social in nature. (4) Employing the behavior modification technique presupposes collection of baseline and treatment data. These principles have been demonstrated to modify behavior in numerous case studies reported by Ullman and Krasner (1965) and Ulrich, Stachnik, and Mabry (1966).

By applying some general principles of behavior to prepare a disturbed deaf child for hearing therapy, the case study described below lends support to using behavior modification techniques in the management of multiply handicapped deaf children.

PROBLEM

Helen M., two years, 10 months old, was diagnosed as having a severe, if not profound, hearing loss. Audiologists at three clinics reported that Helen appeared to have problems in addition to deafness. Such descriptions as these were given: "Helen stares at lights, spins things, looks at her hands, and grinds her teeth almost constantly. She is fascinated by textures. Helen gets very upset when taken into a room and the door is closed. She does not seem very visually alert." On a checklist for diagnosing autism (suggested by Clancy, Dugdale, and Rendle-Short, 1969), the mother and the grandmother, with whom the subject lived, checked 10 out of 14 characteristics as being present.

While she and her mother attended a home demonstration program for parents of deaf children, Helen displayed significant behavior disturbances when her mother or the speech pathologist tried to involve her in activities. Behaviors noted in addition to extreme hyperactivity were screaming, scratching herself, and sometimes vomiting. Hearing therapy and especially a preschool program for the deaf were contraindicated as long as Helen's behavior was not under control. In addition to deafness and an apparent emotional-behavioral disturbance, her attending pediatrician had diagnosed optic nerve damage and an orthopedic problem.

TREATMENT PROGRAM

Because of Helen's multiple problems it was imperative for her program to begin with modifying her maladaptive behaviors so that she could perform in future therapeutic and educational programs.

Planned before treatment began, the two phases of the program were (1) training a team composed of a psychologist, a speech pathologist, and Helen's mother (Mrs. M) how to use behavior principles and (2) implementing those principles to modify Helen's behavior. The speech pathologist and mother were intermediaries between the psychologist and Helen, an approach described by Tharp and Wetzel (1969). The psychologist initially directed Mrs. M and the speech pathologist in behavioral techniques. Including the mother as well as the speech pathologist in the treatment team encouraged consistent use of behavior principles by those mainly involved with Helen in her therapeutic program and in her home. Helen clearly would need more behavioral work than could be handled in a clinical situation; training the mother for several treatment roles would facilitate her learning to use behavioral principles so that she could maximize generalization of appropriate behaviors at home. Much of the training was for the mother's benefit—her being a member of the treatment team encouraged her to feel on an equal level with the speech pathologist and psychologist in her child's treatment. Her interest in active participation was considered to be maintained throughout the treatment period. There were two treatment sessions weekly.

Phase 1

Four steps were taken to train the psychologist, the speech pathologist and Mrs. M for their roles:

1. Each team member read *Living with Children*, by Patterson and Gullion (1968); some unpublished materials that William Bricker, of George Peabody College for Teachers, Nashville, Tennessee, adapted from the work of Ogden Lindsley; and two case studies by Ulrich, Stachnik, and Mabry (1966). They viewed the film "Teaching the Mentally Retarded: A Positive Approach," produced by the Southern Region Educational Board.

2. The three team members met to discuss the foregoing information in relation to Helen's behavior.

3. The psychologist taught the speech pathologist and Mrs. M how to operate a signaling device used to cue the person working with Helen and a recording device used to record Helen's behavior during treatment.

4. In the beginning of treatment the psychologist, the speech pathologist, and Mrs. M alternated as the signaler (the one cuing the therapist), the observer-data recorder, and the therapist to learn the roles played in Helen's treatment.

Phase 2

These steps were used to modify Helen's behavior:

1. As long as Helen screamed, the therapist completely ignored her by turning away. As soon as Helen stopped screaming, the therapist reinforced her

by turning to her, patting her, and saying, "That's good, Helen." The therapist's ignoring was withdrawal of positive reinforcement, and the therapist's attention was positive reinforcement contingent upon the desired behavior of ceasing to scream.

2. After screaming was eliminated, the same procedure was used to begin to shape Helen's attending behavior, attending being defined here as staying physically close to the therapist.

3. To shape the terminal behavior desired, that of sitting in a chair beside the therapist and performing tasks presented for at least 15 minutes, milk shake or coke and social praise were used as reinforcement, intermittently throughout the period of sitting.

4. During the first weeks of treatment Mrs. M was required to keep records of Helen's screaming behavior at home. Time-out periods, putting Helen in a bedroom stripped of toys each time she began to scream when not getting her way and leaving her there for two minutes after she stopped screaming, were used to help eliminate crying at home.

Baseline Data

The baseline data (Figures 5.1-5.4) were obtained by the speech patholo-gist and the evaluating psychologist. For three sessions Helen ran around the room crying or screaming an average of 96% (Figure 5.1) of the approximate 20-minute sessions, approaching the therapist at the work table an average of only 4% (Figure 5.2). Sitting and attending to tasks presented to her were absent (Figures 5.3 and 5.4).

Treatment Data

The treatment results were considered reliable. To effect accurate data collection, the psychologist and speech pathologist initially alternated between the roles of therapist and observer-data recorder, with Mrs. M serving as observer-data recorder only. When Mrs. M acted as therapist, the psychologist was signaler and the speech pathologist, data recorder. In Sessions 12 through 34 both the speech pathologist, who was therapist, and Mrs. M, the observer-data recorder, collected data. In addition, many sessions throughout the treatment period were videotaped, allowing the psychologist to check the data collected.

In figure 5.1 the percentage of time Helen spent crying is indicated on the ordinate and the treatment sessions on the abscissa. With the behavior modification technique described in Treatment Step 1, that is, completely ignoring Helen as long as she screamed and giving attention to her when she stopped screaming, Helen's screaming decreased from 96% in the baseline sessions to 0% in Treatment Session 5. With screaming eliminated, the

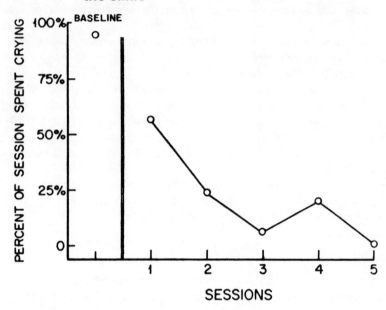

FIGURE 5.1. Modification of screaming and crying behavior at the clinic

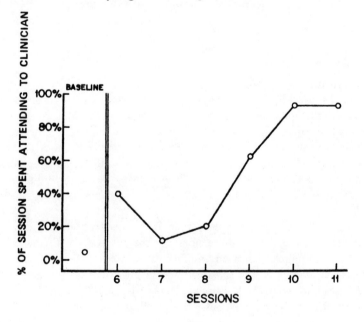

FIGURE 5.2. Shaping attending behavior

therapist began to reinforce Helen for attending to him, or approaching and staying close to him.

Figure 5.2 indicates that Helen's attending increased from 40% in Treatment Session 6 to 95% in Sessions 10 and 11. The team then felt that Helen could realistically be encouraged to sit in a chair beside the therapist and perform tasks presented to her.

Helen's progress in Sessions 12 through 23 is plotted in Figure 5.3. For illustration, the 12 sessions were collapsed into six blocks of two sessions each. The percentage of the session Helen sat and attended to tasks is represented on the ordinate. The tasks presented were tasks simple for Helen, such as stringing beads and putting rings on a stick. While Helen sat and performed, she was reinforced intermittently, not only with the usual social praise but also with sips of milk shake or coke, which had been determined to be powerful reinforcers in her natural environment. Helen was allowed to get out of her chair but was reinforced only as long as she attended to tasks while sitting. When she refused to sit, she was ignored and was not allowed to play with any task items. By Sessions 22 and 23, during which Helen sat with the therapist 96% and 93% of the sessions, the team felt that she could be required

FIGURE 5.3.   Establishing sitting behavior

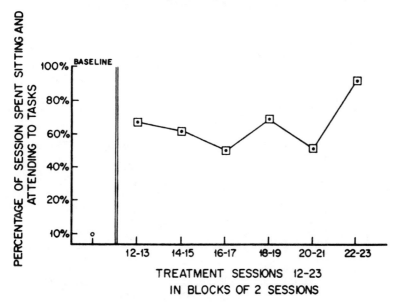

to sit continuously, with an attempt to increase the continuous seated time to a desirable length for a hearing therapy program.

Figure 5.4 indicates continuous time Helen sat and performed simple tasks presented to her from Sessions 24 through 34. On the ordinate are indicated the minutes during which Helen sat and performed continuously. At this time, when Helen exhibited pronounced restlessness, the session ended after she performed one or more item presented to her. The time increased from seven minutes in Session 24 to 14 minutes in Session 31. Although Helen missed a month of treatment between Sessions 28 and 29 because of corrective orthopedic surgery, her continuous performance decreased by only one minute. In Session 32 hearing therapy activities were begun. While her attention span was still short, she could be required to perform in auditory training and matching activities and to look at the therapist's face. By that time Helen's main reinforcement was social praise and items with which she performed a structured activity, with coke used only intermittently. In addition, both of her parents were able to play semistructured games requiring shape and color matching with Helen for approximately 30 continuous minutes daily.

FIGURE 5.4. Increasing continuous sitting time

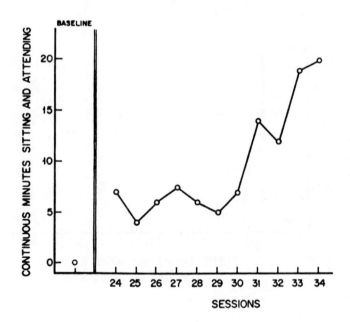

FIGURE 5.5. Modification of screaming behavior at home

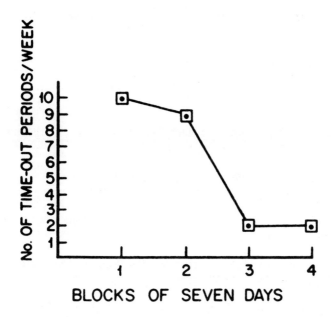

Mrs. M's being a member of the treatment team was considered crucial in effecting Helen's behavior changes. In the beginning, Mrs. M was taught to reinforce desirable behavior and to ignore undesirable behavior. When crying was being extinguished in sessions at the clinic, Mrs. M kept records of Helen's screaming behavior at home. As part of her training, she served as therapist in several treatment sessions, with the psychologist and speech pathologist observing, and she participated as observer data-recorder throughout the other sessions. That Helen's continuous performance decreased by only one minute after missing a month of treatment was believed to be attributable to Mrs. M's implementing treatment principles at home.

Figure 5.5 is an example of Mrs. M's using time-out periods to help eliminate Helen's screaming behavior at home. Each block on the abscissa represents seven days. The number of time-outs, represented on the ordinate, decreased from 10 in the first week of treatment to two in the third and fourth weeks. Mrs. M's reaction to being a team member in Helen's treatment was positive. She commented from time to time that her training before Helen's treatment and her participation helped her to modify other behaviors at home. One outstanding behavior Mrs. M herself brought under control was Helen's feeding problem.

REFERENCES

Clancy, H., Dugdale, A., and Rendle-Short, J., The diagnosis of infantile autism. *Develpm. Med. Child Neurol.*, II, 432-442 (1969).

Ladson, M. R., The education of emotionally handicapped deaf children. *Proceedings of the 42nd Meeting of the Convention of American Instructors of the Deaf. Amer. Instr. Deaf*, 42. Washington, D.C.: U.S. Govt. Printing Off., 115-119 (1965).

Lennan, R. K., Report on a program for emotionally disturbed deaf boys. *Amer. Ann. Deaf*, 115, 469-480 (1970).

Patterson, G. R., and Gullion, M. E., *Living with Children: New Methods for Parents and Teachers*. Champaign, Ill.: Research Press (1968).

Salzinger, K., Behavior theory and problems of the deaf. *Amer. Ann. Deaf*, 115, 459-468 (1970).

Tharp, R. G., and Wetzel, R. J., *Behavior Modification in the Natural Environment*. New York: Academic Press (1969).

Ullman, L., and Krasner, L. (Eds.), *Case Studies in Behavior Modification*. New York: Holt, Rinehart (1965).

Ulrich, R., Stachnik, T., and Mabry, J. (Eds.), *Control of Human Behavior*. Glenview, Ill.: Scott, Foresman (1966).

Warren, S. A., Setting our sights for the emotionally disturbed deaf. *Proceedings of the 40th Meeting of the Convention of the American Instructors of the Deaf. Amer. Instr. Deaf*, 42. Washington, D.C.: U.S. Govt. Printing Off., 71-74 (1961).

Withrow, F. B., Acquisition of language by deaf children with other disabilities. *Volta Rev.*, 68, 106-115 (1966).

6

SPEECH

INTRODUCTION

Influenced by Skinner's work (1957), Ferster (1961) published one of the first papers on the application of operant learning principles to language acquisition of autistic children. Lovaas et al. (1966) published their work with 11 severely disturbed children, emphasizing the use of immediate punishment (spanking and shouting) to suppress stereotypical repetitive motor behavior, followed by immediate reward (candy, physical contact, and social praise), cueing and fading responses, along with successive approximation to teach language and social competencies. The following year, Risley and Wolf (1967) reported the use of nonphysical punishers ("time-out"). With certain cases, physical restraint and isolation have proved helpful in reducing disruptive and distracting behaviors.

The articles selected in this chapter provide some of the first examples of systems of language training. Stark, Rosenbaum, Schwartz, and Wisan (1973) describe the principles and procedures for language acquisition of nonverbal children. Particular attention is paid to the underlying principles of data collection and analysis, and to the modification of antecedent and consequent events in social interaction. They carefully outline a three-month outpatient and home training program for beginning language acquisition. In the following section, Hartung (1970) presents an excellent review of procedures for the establishment of functional speech with autistic children.

Stuttering

Among verbally deficient children, stuttering has been an area of major clinical and research attention. Stuttering occurs in about 1 to 2 percent of school age children (Bakwin & Bakwin, 1972). It spontaneously disappears in 80 percent of cases and has little relationship to behavior problems, neurotic symptomology, or other psychiatric disorders in parents. Johnson (1959) believes that normal dysfluencies lead to stuttering due to the negative reactions of others. Quarrington (1974), in a review of the literature, finds parents of stutterers to be submissive and more tolerant of speech and behavioral deviations than other parents. Stuttering is considered by some (Brutten & Shoemaker, 1967) to be acquired by classical conditioning and maintained by the operant behaviors associated with it. Despite a number of theories, little direct evidence exists to support any of them.

Behavioral approaches to treatment have emphasized desensitization (Lanyon, 1969) and other anxiety reduction procedures, and a number of seemingly unrelated techniques such as the use of speech making and white noise (Gruber, 1971), shadowing (Kondas, 1967), various rhythm techniques using a metronome (Brady, 1971), delayed auditory feedback (Goldiamond, 1965), and various other methods (Webster, 1977).

Kondas (1967), for example, building on the work of Cherry and Sayers (1956), demonstrated the influence of shadowing on speech fluency in 19 stammerers between 5 and 20 years of age. The shadowing technique involves graduated practice in repeating exactly what was just read by the therapist. Kondas trained children both in the clinic and the home.

Goldiamond (1965) has pioneered the use of delayed auditory feedback (DAF) speech dysfluencies. DAF is initially used in structured reading to decrease stuttering to the point that a slow fluent speech is produced. Its use is then faded and the rate of fluent speech is slowly accelerated, first in the clinic and then in a variety of natural settings.

Starkweather (1973), in a behavioral analysis of Van Riper's (1972) therapy for stutterers, illustrates the use of behavioral techniques within the context of traditional speech therapy. In the first phase of Van Riper's "symptomatic therapy," he attempts to create a permissive atmosphere that accepts, even encourages, stuttering. The second phase involves experimental assignments in which children stutter most. In the third phase, the therapist begins to focus on stress situations. Patients are directed to seek out situations of increasing stressfulness to allow their children to develop higher and higher tolerances of stress. Out of this grows a confidence on the part of stutterers that they have control over their stuttering. Once this procedure is established, various techniques are used to teach effortless, nonstruggling speech. Patients are taught first to repeat each word in a nonstruggled manner but purposefully to stutter; this process is called cancellation. Later, stutterers are taught to relax their speech in the middle of a speech blockage, continuing to shift the relaxation to the beginning of the blockage and eventually to the cues associated with stuttering.

Webster (1977) developed a "Precision Fluency Shaping Program" for the treatment of stutterers, which emphasizes precise analysis and restructuring of the stutterer's speech patterns, using carefully defined, small, progressive steps. This program provides intensive and systematic training in how clients physically form sounds, syllables, words, and sentences. Emphasis on the fine details of articulation and voicing produces fluent speech. To gain precision of control over voice onsets, Webster uses a small computer, the voice monitor, to measure voice onset characteristics and to provide training in "gentle onset" of voice. Also given is instruction in breath control.

Brady (1971) has developed the use of metronome-conditioned speech retraining (MCSR) in the treatment of severe stuttering. He trains his patients with a desk metronome to relax and to slow speech to the point that it is highly fluent. The rate is then gradually increased to approximate normal speech. Acknowledging problems in shifting from speaking with a metronome to speaking without one, Brady describes the use of a miniaturized electronic metronome that can be worn behind the ear like a hearing aid. This metronome can then be used in public settings without ready detection as an aid to transition from the clinic to the natural setting. All these methods offer specific techniques that are relatively effective in gaining behavioral control over the stuttering behavior. Unfortunately, many of these techniques are elaborate, laboratory-based procedures that do not easily transfer to the natural environment.

Azrin and Nunn (1974) describe the use of the "Habit Reversal Procedure," a technique that has been widely applied to common nervous habits, for the treatment of stuttering. Their basic strategy is to have the patient interrupt speech at points of anticipated stuttering, as well as natural pause points, and to continue speaking after breathing and pausing, which are regarded as behaviors incompatible with stuttering. Patients are trained in relaxation, stimulus control techniques, contingency management, and self-management. In addition to laboratory training, patients are expected to practice at home, and family support is encouraged. This article provides an excellent example of a clinically useful, multimodal treatment procedure that can be used by the practicing clinician without elaborate clinical tools and settings.

References

Azrin, N. H., & Nunn, R. G. A rapid method of eliminating stuttering by regulated breathing approach. *Behaviour Research and Therapy*, 1974, *12*, 279-286.

Bakwin, H. & Bakwin, R. M. *Behavior Disorders in Children.* Philadelphia: W. B. Saunders, 1972.

Brady, J. P. Metronome-conditioned speech retraining for stuttering. *Behavior Therapy*, 1971, *2*, 129-150.

Brutten, E. J., & Shoemaker, D. J. *The modification of stuttering.* Englewood Cliffs, N.J.: Prentice Hall, 1967.

Cherry, C., & Sayers, B. McA. Experiments upon the total inhibition of stammering by external control and some clinical results. *Journal of Psychosomatic Research*, 1956, *1*, 233-246.

Ferster, C. B. Positive reinforcement and behavioral deficits of autistic children. *Child Development*, 1961, *32*, 437-456.

Goldiamond, I. Stuttering and fluency as manipulable operant classes. In L. Krasner & L. P. Ullmann (Eds.), *Research in behavior modification: New developments and implications.* New York: Holt, Rinehart & Winston, 1965.

Gruber, L. The use of portable voice masker in stuttering therapy. *Journal of Speech and Hearing Disorders*, 1971, *36*, 287-289.

Hartung, J. R. A review of procedures to increase verbal imitation skills and functional speech in autistic children. *Journal of Speech and Hearing Disorders*, 1970, *35*, 203-217.

Johnson, W. *The onset of stuttering: Research findings and implications.* Minneapolis: University of Minnesota Press, 1959.

Kondas, O. The treatment of stammering in children by the shadowing method. *Behaviour Research and Therapy*, 1967, *5*, 325-329.

Lanyon, R. I. Behavior change in stuttering through systematic desensitization. *Journal of Speech and Hearing Disorders*, 1969, *34*, 253-260.

Lovaas, O. I., Berberich, J. P., Perloff, B. F., & Schaeffer, B. Acquisition of imitative speech in schizophrenic children. *Science*, 1966, *151*, 705-707.

Quarrington, B. The parents of stuttering children: The literature re-examined. *Canadian Psychiatric Association Journal*, 1974, *19*, 103-110.

Risley, T., & Wolf, M. Establishing functional speech in echolalic children. *Behaviour Research and Therapy*, 1967, *5*, 73-88.

Sanok, R. L., & Striefel, S. Elective mutism: Generalization of verbal responding across people in settings. *Behavior Therapy*, 1979, *10*, 357-371.

Skinner, B. F. *Verbal behavior.* New York: Appleton, 1957.

Stark, J., Rosenbaum, R. L., Schwartz, D., & Wisan, A. The nonverbal child: Some clinical guidelines. *Journal of Speech and Hearing Disorders*, 1973, *38*, 59-72.

Starkweather, C. W. A behavioral analysis of Van Riperian therapy for stutterers. *Journal of Communication Disorders*, 1973, *6*, 273-291.

Van Riper, C. G. *Speech correction: Principles and methods* (5th ed.). Englewood Cliffs, N.J.: Prentice Hall, 1972.

Webster, R. L. A few observations on the manipulation of speech response characteristics in stutterers. *Journal of Communication Disorders* 1977, *10*, 73-76.

THE NONVERBAL CHILD:
SOME CLINICAL GUIDELINES

Joel Stark
Robert L. Rosenbaum
Dorothea Schwartz
Arlene Wisan

This article describes some principles and procedures related to language training for nonverbal children. Reinforcement theory is discussed and illustrative cases are presented. Emphasis is on the application of an experimental approach to the modification of language behavior. The role of recent research in language acquisition as well as the relationship of the language training to the social environment is questioned and discussed.

The establishment of adequate language performance in the young nonverbal child is a complex and arduous task. The purpose of this article is to describe some of the procedures we have been using with the nonverbal child. In the first part, we will outline some of the principles upon which we base our work. This is followed by case studies illustrating the application of these principles and a discussion of some relevant questions about the direction of our therapeutic procedures.

BEHAVIOR OF THE CHILDREN

The children with whom we are concerned have very limited functional communication. They are between three and six years of age and are enrolled

Reprinted from *Journal of Speech and Hearing Disorders*, 1973, *38*, 59-71. Copyright 1973 by the American Speech, Language and Hearing Society. Reprinted by permission.

Joel Stark, Robert L. Rosenbaum, Dorothea Schwartz, and Arlene Wisan are at Queens College of the City University of New York, Flushing, New York.

at the clinic for a minimum of three hours of individual therapy per week. The language behaviors of these children vary considerably. Some have never been heard to produce speech and are "nonverbal" in the truest sense. Others echo utterances without regard for communicative intent. Some of the children are able to imitate vocal and nonvocal stimuli and may respond appropriately to language where the referent is present and the form is simple (for example, "Sit down," "Give me the ball").

For most of the children, the possibility of some type of central nervous system dysfunction was considered the primary etiological factor. Based upon observation of performance with nonverbal tasks such as block building, sorting, and puzzles, there was evidence to suggest that these children possess enough intellectual integrity to learn verbal language. Many of the children have behavioral patterns which are asocial and which have been found to occur in the histories of children classified as autistic, aphasic, and brain-injured. They often do not look at people; they cry frequently, play with toys in a bizarre manner, smile and laugh inappropriately, bite their hands and arms and move about the room randomly. Gaining control of their behavior so that they will attend to the stimuli being presented by the clinician is often the first major goal in their training.

UNDERLYING PRINCIPLES

There are some constructs which guide us in our work with the nonverbal child. Among the most significant are: (1) Language behavior is composed of observable and recordable events. (2) The nature and frequency of language behavior is affected by what happens before and after the behavior is emitted.

Thus, we are concerned with the character of the discriminative stimulus (S^D) in the presence of which a response is reinforced, as well as with the reinforcing stimulus (S^R), which is functionally related to the response it follows.

Recording Progress

It is difficult for clinicians to collect data as they do therapy, since the use of checklists, manual counters, and other such recording devices may interfere with the presentation of stimuli. The use of audio and videotape recorders removes much of the initial recording burden from clinicians, but requires time-consuming transcription at some later time. In addition, this equipment is very expensive. In university clinics such as ours, students are often available to record relevant behaviors during the therapy session. Ideally, the recording of behaviors of interest would be fully automated; however, the development of transducers for speech behaviors has been slow.

In many programs, therapeutic progress is measured by administering pre- and posttest instruments. This affords an adequate means for charting progress over periods of time, but is of little value in the day-to-day management of the child. We have found it exceedingly useful to gather data daily in the course of therapy and to use these data as a means of monitoring the effectiveness of our procedures. Thus, when a clinician attempts to teach a language skill to a child, there is a record of the number of times the stimuli were presented, under what conditions, and with what success. The clinician is able to modify whatever procedures need to be modified on the basis of empirical observation rather than subjective speculation.

The Appendix to this paper shows one of the recording forms which we have found useful. For each trial, the discriminative stimulus in the presence of which the child is expected to respond is noted. Thus, if the clinician held up a picture or an object and said, "What's this?" the picture and the clinician's question would be recorded in this column. In the next four columns, checks are used. *Pro* refers to whether or not the clinicians had to prompt or aid the child in order for him to respond. For example, she may produce the first phoneme of the response she wants the child to emit, or help the child to close his lips to produce a sound. *Mod* is a form of prompt where the clinician or another person demonstrates the desired response for the child. In the R column, the clinician records the response. The S^R refers to the reinforcing stimulus. If the child's response was followed by a token, social praise, food, or any other reinforcer, this is checked. The last column permits the observer to record any novel behavior or to comment on the trial. This form is organized in blocks of 10 trials to simplify summarizing the data. In spite of the limitations, we have found this recording procedure to be an invaluable adjunct in our therapy.

We should add a word of caution here regarding what could appear to be a simplistic way of looking at the process of language therapy. Certainly more happens when two people sit across a table in the clinic than can possibly be recorded on a form like this. Apart from the need to devise forms to record different behaviors, clinicians must be continually aware of the many variables which can influence progress. These include the verbal behavior emitted by clinicians before and after stimuli are presented; the latency of the responses; the visual, auditory, and tactile-kinesthetic dimensions of the stimuli; and changes in the physical environment.

Experimental Approaches

Data collection and analysis does often demonstrate that we have made improvement in therapy. More recent case reports have described progress by keeping careful records of the subjects' responses (Goldstein and Lanyon, 1971; Leonard, 1971; Ryan, 1971; Daly et al., 1972). However, one might argue that, in some instances, maturation and the passage of time might have the same effect. Hence, a major responsibility is to apply experimental procedures to study some of the variables responsible for the modification of behavior. That is, to examine causal relationships and demonstrate that a specific procedure was or was not instrumental in producing change. To this end, the clinical experimental procedures reported by McReynolds and Huston (1971) and Shaw and Shrum (1972) are especially instructive.

One experimental design which is commonly used is referred to as a *reversal* design or an A-B-A procedure. The clinician first observes and records the child's behavior under standard conditions, and this is referred to as a *baseline*. During the next few sessions, we may begin an experimental procedure of some kind, while continuing to record the child's behavioral responses. Perhaps we will change the reinforcer or the reinforcement schedule, vary the nature of the discriminative stimulus by using a model, or a different kind of prompt, or different stimuli. After the experimental treatment sessions, we then return to the baseline condition to see if the behavior remains when the experimental variables are removed. This reversal allows us to verify, in a more precise way, whether or not our procedures are responsible for changes in behavior.

Another design is referred to as a *multiple baseline* design. Here, more than one behavior is recorded during the baseline condition. However, in the experimental conditions only one of these behaviors is trained at a time to determine whether the experimental treatment is effective. There are, of course, many possible variations to these experimental procedures.

THE USE OF CONSEQUENCES

The application of a reinforcing stimuli to gain control of behavior can best be illustrated by some clinical studies. Barry (chronological age four years) moved about the room in a circular motion, at times touching and smelling the walls and furniture. He did not respond in the presence of stimuli such as "Barry sit" or other verbal stimuli intended to have him look at the clinician. His mother reported that he was generally unaware of the presence of people. At home he would not eat at the table, sit on a chair, or play with toys. During the year, a number of ritualistic behaviors emerged, including head banging, skin biting, repetitive circular movement, and sucking of a knuckle.

After we observed Barry's behavior, our first goal was to get him to attend to the clinician. At first we wanted him to sit in a chair. Since he did sit on a toilet seat at home, teaching him sitting behavior seemed feasible. The sitting response in the presence of the discriminative stimulus "Barry sit" was modeled by the clinicians. Then we prompted Barry by placing him in the chair and reinforcing this with social praise, bubbles, and candy. His inappropriate and disruptive behavior continued for three hour-long sessions and he failed to respond to the "sit down" stimulus. During the third session, there were only three correct unprompted responses out of 54 trials.

Because Barry's mother reported that he especially enjoyed eating bacon, during the fourth session the clinician placed a piece of bacon on the chair. Barry remained close to the chair, although he still would not sit down. The clinician then held the bacon in front of the chair. As Barry moved in line with the chair, she said, "Barry, sit," placed him in the chair, and gave him a piece of bacon. During this session, Barry responded, without having to be prompted, 21 times out of 46 presentations of the discriminative stimulus. By the seventh session there was 100% correct responding to more than 20 presentations of the discriminative stimulus. We continued to present nonvocal and vocal stimuli for Barry to imitate and found that when the bacon was removed, the latency of Barry's responses increased from an average of two seconds to more than 10 seconds. In addition, most of the responses were not accurate. As soon as the bacon was re-presented, the nature and frequency of his responding increased. Hence, the clinician found an effective reinforcing stimulus.

Sometimes clinicians are naive about the way they describe and use reinforcers. The fact that a child is being fed, or is given a piece of candy or a trinket, and fails to respond any differently is often used as evidence that the application of reinforcement principles is not effective. Clearly, the successful application of a consequent event or reinforcing stimulus is highly individual. The effectiveness of such an event or stimulus can only be measured by examining subsequent changes in the behavior which it follows. The search for an effective reinforcing stimulus, particularly for the nonverbal child, is a difficult one. Clinicians need to find out about the objects and routines which produce observable changes in behavior at home. How do the parents teach, discipline, love, and in the broadest sense, live with the child? While social praise in its many forms is the most conventional reinforcer, it alone may not modify the behavior of the young nonverbal child.

Use of Tokens

As Girardeau and Spradlin (1970) point out, a token system is potentially the most useful reinforcer in therapy. The advantage of the token system is that it does not interfere with the child's response. The clinician need not wait until the child chews and swallows a piece of food before presenting the next stimulus. Tokens can be presented or withdrawn (for example, response cost); they allow the child to earn the kind of object or activity which is most reinforcing for him; and they permit the use of more powerful reinforcers (such as a trip to a zoo or restaurant, or a highly desired toy).

However, for most nonverbal children, it is not possible to delay the delivery of a reinforcer over a long period. The opportunity to exchange the tokens needs to be afforded often.

In one study, we examined the child's responses contingent upon social praise (for example, "Good boy") and a token system where he could earn a piece of food or candy for every three tokens he received. (See Figure 6.1.) In Sessions 1 through 3 and 8 through 11, we used a token for food exchange, and in Sessions 4 through 7, social praise alone was used. There was a significant difference in the percentage of correct responding when the token exchange system was used. The child did significantly more poorly when only social praise was the reinforcer.

Often reinforcers are special for a specific child and we have studied them. Because of space limitations, we will present anecdotal accounts rather than describe the experimental procedures in detail. Neil (CA 3.5) had no functional speech, did not respond to people moving about or to his parents leaving the room. He avoided eye to face contact. When the examiner carried him, bounced him, swung him, threw him into the air and caught him, or even tickled him, his only response was a gentle attempt to escape. An outstanding ability was his "reading" of letters and numbers. The clinician would write these letters and numbers and Neil was able to say them. As he walked down

FIGURE 6.1. Responses to therapy using different reinforcers

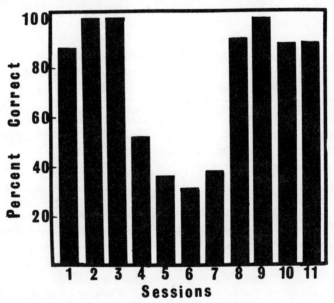

In Sessions 1-4 and 8-11, social praise and a token system were used. In Sessions 4-7, social praise alone was used.

the hall he would read the numbers on each of the clinic doors. To return him to the waiting room, the clinician would take a plastic letter, hold it in front of her, and walk down the hall, at which time Neil would follow. The efficacy of plastic letters as a reinforcing stimulus in gaining control of his behavior and strengthening his language performance was studied. We presented the discriminative stimuli in blocks of 10 trials during part of three consecutive sessions, alternating between a social reinforcer plus a plastic letter and social reinforcement alone. While Neil's overall percentage of correct responding did not differ significantly during these experimental treatments, the discriminative stimuli had to be presented at least twice as often when only social reinforcers were used. Neil was not as attentive or interested in the task. When the letters were used, he made responses immediately.

One child's behavior was not being maintained with food reinforcers. Jerry (CA five) would play with the food and then bite his hands. Although saying, "No, don't do that," would be effective at times, this did not increase the number of correct responses substantially, nor did it decrease his hand biting. Jerry may have been reinforced by the attention given him when he played with his food and was told to eat it. Therefore, a different type of reinforcing stimulus was arranged. We instituted a play area physically apart from the work table area. A simple sorting task was presented. Jerry merely had to place a block in a box. When Jerry put it in or imitated the modeling clinician, he was taken to the play area for a two-minute period. At the sixth trial Jerry reached for the block even before he sat down. Then the clinician presented the discriminative stimulus two times before allowing him to go to the play area. At the ninth trial, the clinician called him to the work area instead of taking his hand. At the sixteenth trial he had to respond correctly three times before play was allowed. At the twenty-fifth trial, there were four correct responses. At the twenty-ninth trial, he walked back to the clinician, and by the thirty-third trial he ran back to the work area from the play area. At this point Jerry was required to produce five consecutive correct responses before reinforcement. During the next session, the task was changed to include discrimination between blocks of different colors and shapes, and the play period was decreased in time. The discriminative stimuli were gradually made more difficult and the reinforcement schedule was altered so that the time spent in the play area was decreased. Within eight sessions, Jerry was working effectively in blocks of 20 trials where the response was followed by social praise. At the end of a block of 20 trials, he was permitted to go to the play area.

Alan (CA 3.11) had no functional speech, threw objects which were within his reach, and never engaged in conventional children's play activities. He would neither sit on his mother's lap nor in a chair. He usually held and smelled his blanket while having to be carried from one place to another. Alan cried frequently and often scratched his flesh; his body was covered with scratches. His parents had to keep long-sleeved shirts and heavier pants on him so that he would not bleed from the scratching.

When we first saw Alan, we recorded the number of times that he began to cry and the amount of crying he did during these initial sessions. From the outset we introduced a time out from positive reinforcement procedure. Whenever Alan began to cry the clinician turned to the side and removed any stimulus materials and reinforcers which were present until five seconds after this undesirable behavior ceased. Because some of his undesirable behavior may have been maintained by the adults who were attending to him, we removed all reinforcers whenever Alan became disruptive. The amount of crying was significantly modified by the fourth week. Compared to the first week, when Alan cried 30% of the time (56 crying starts), by the fourteenth week, he cried only 0.06% of the time.

Some of these procedures were introduced at home. Of interest was the fact that when Alan banged his head on the floor at home, he would go to where there was an area rug and bang his head on that rather than on the bare floor. His parents responded to the head banging by yelling, "No." and, "Stop." and this had little success. We advised his mother to ignore this behavior, and within a month it ceased, except in the presence of his father, who continued to attend to it. When his father also began to ignore the behavior, it stopped. Many nonverbal children may use deviant behaviors to control their environment.

In selecting a consequent event, we are sometimes limited only by our own imagination. We have variously used hugging, tickling, jumping, rocking, balloon popping, trinkets, water play, flashing lights, and a variety of foods, including ice cream and soda. What is important is that the selection and application of consequences be derived from empirical observation of the behavior.

ANTECEDENT EVENTS

We have been emphasizing some of the ways a child's behavior can be brought under stimulus control and maintained so that clinicians can more effectively teach him. Now we are concerned with the kinds of discriminative stimuli which should be presented in therapy. Which stimuli should be presented first? Can you teach specific language responses or do you merely devise ways to unlock the child's "innate capacity for using language"? What are the contributions of the different theoretical approaches on which the clinician bases his daily goals?

Most studies of child language are observational in nature and have been concerned with the production of language. Typically, spontaneous utterances of children are collected in a naturalistic setting such as the home, and then these are analyzed. Investigators found that children who began to use two-word utterances possessed grammars which were uniquely childlike. One small class of words occurred frequently in a relatively fixed position, while others with which they were combined occurred less frequently. Braine (1963) called these "pivot" and "x-words"; Brown and Bellugi (1964), "functors" and "contentives"; Miller and Erwin (1964), "operators" and "nonoperators." Bloom (1970, 1971) raised some important objections to the application of these "pivot" grammars. She felt that the semantic basis was overlooked and showed that the child used the same grammatical construction to mean different things. For example, "Mommy sock" may designate the possessor, be a request to have her socks put on, or be a description of her mother putting on socks. While the categorization of speech events in terms of their function is not new, we have found Bloom's categories more useful than Skinner's (1957) and most others. She classified utterances as follows:

1. Comments occurred when the referent was manifest and functioned to name or point out objects, persons, or events. A comment does not attempt to influence the behavior of the receiver (for example, "That's a car").
2. Reports occurred in the absence of a receiver and were informative utterances directed to a receiver. Reports do not attempt to influence the behavior of the receiver (for example, "I have a car" [at home]).
3. Directions were characterized by the child's seeking a change in the context, which he is unable or unwilling to effect himself, involving the behavior of someone else (for example, "Give me the car").
4. Questions were characterized by the child's seeking information or confirmation and were directed to a receiver (for example, "Is that your car?").

The implications of an approach which emphasizes the function of a speech event may be important for modifying the language of nonverbal children. Language responses occur within a communication interaction, and it is the child's success in communication which is the relevant measure of his progress in the clinic. Hence, clinicians must transcend the highly structured and artificial setting of the clinic and be able to transfer these responses to more naturalistic and functional settings. Perhaps if clinicians would use certain kinds of speech events with a child, it would accelerate the acquisition process. An even more urgent question which clinicians must answer relates to the complexity of the language forms which they use when talking to a child. Should clinicians reduce the complexity of their own speech? Should they omit connectives, articles, and other redundant parts of an utterance? Clinicians need to consider the paucity of language which many nonverbal children have and modify their own language so that utterances can be responded to appropriately.

With regard to the formulation of specific teaching programs, we can only hypothesize that if children are taken through a prescribed series of steps which are consistent with the normal sequence, they will develop functional language. To this end, a number of systematic programs have been reported (Lovaas, 1968; Bricker and Bricker, 1970; Hartung, 1970). The programming hierarchy includes the acquisition of imitative skills at the outset and the gradual shaping of responses. By pairing the vocal imitation with objects, the child learns a core of noun labels. In the presence of the object, the vocal imitation produces reinforcement. Hence, the object becomes a discriminative stimulus for the response. These responses are expanded into longer utterances by combining the objects with carrier phrases such as "Give me _____" or "I want _____." Presumably, the language responses become functional for the child.

These programs are well-intentioned and do produce positive results. Perhaps their major function is to establish the conditions for further growth. The child begins to respond to verbal stimuli and is reinforced in their presence. The hope is that he will seek new ways to use language and make continued progress.

A significant question for clinicians who work with nonverbal children is the degree to which they can apply the findings of researchers working in normal language acquisition. Does the nonverbal child need to pass through certain stages in the developmental sequence? How does the establishment of imitative skills relate to language behavior? Do these children require special training in perceptual skills (such as visual and auditory memory and visual-motor sequencing)? How are these skills related to the acquisition of verbal language? What experiences provide the cognitive basis for language behavior?

In spite of the many teaching procedures in the literature, there is much more that we do not know about the acquisition of language in the nonverbal child than there is that we do know. The important criterion is the degree to which we measure the effectiveness of our procedures and continue to search for new approaches.

Research in normal language acquisition is providing some significant guidelines. Bloom (1971) has pointed out that the earliest syntactic utterances are related to existence, nonexistence, and action upon a referent. Hence, programs designed to establish language in the nonverbal child might attend to what we call *verbing*. Children experience the relations between people (agents), objects, and actions well before they learn attributes of objects. They may respond in the presence of "red ball" but the response will be specific to that particular red ball. It may be more appropriate to consider the action involved and to program a series of stimuli which present relations between actions with people and objects. Instead of modifier-noun constructions, clinicians need to present stimuli which relate to the world of action. Thus, they can teach "More car," "No car," "Push car," or "Car go" rather than "Red car" or "Big car." Similarly, an attempt to establish morphological distinctions such as plurals or different tense endings should be delayed until much later in the program. The basic question for the clinician is what or who are the [people, objects] doing.

Programming Stimuli

We have often found it helpful to use the construct of "critical elements" in organizing stimulus materials. Functionally, these are the objects, agents, actions, and attributes which constitute the different parts of a sentence. Clinicians should manipulate only one element at a time. For example, in the presence of a picture and the verbal S^D "What is the man doing?" the child would emit, "Sitting." The clinician would then present opportunities for discriminated responding to the actions or the agents, but not both. The clinician would either program verbs and present pictures of men throwing, walking, running, eating, and so on or use the same action verb and change the agent. Once each word class has been responded to appropriately, action-agent units (for example, Who is doing what?) may be introduced.

As we have pointed out earlier, there are many variables involved in the presentation of stimuli, and careful programming demands that we take little for granted. With a child whom we are teaching to respond in the presence of particular objects, we first need to have him emit a response in the presence of one object. At the outset, the clinician might say, "Give me the [object]," and reinforce the child when he picks it up. Or he may modify the procedure by presenting an outstretched hand as he says, "Give me," or prompting initial responses by taking the child's hand and moving it toward the object. Once appropriate responding in the presence of one object has been achieved, the clinician may place two objects on the table, changing their position randomly and reinforcing the child only when he responds appropriately to the verbal S^Ds. This procedure can be extended using additional objects and gradually increasing the child's repertoire. Sometimes, different features of the S^D must be intensified or modified to insure correct responding. Clinicians may speak louder, or use larger or different visual materials, and depending upon the kind of stimuli presented, reinforce successive approximations to the desired response.

Building as much success as possible into the teaching program is essential. At the outset, we have often found it more advisable to use nonverbal stimuli such as geometric shapes for the child to match or gross motor movements for the child to imitate. Gradually, these can be paired with a verbal S^D. For example, the child may learn standing behavior in the presence of the clinician who models it and reinforces the child when he stands. After this, the verbal S^D "Stand" is added and the child responds in the presence of the model and the verbal S^D. Before long the child will respond in the presence of the verbal S^D alone.

There are many different ways to present stimuli, and too often clinicians fail to rely upon visual and tactile kinesthetic cues. With one child, we used large sheets of differently colored construction paper to assist him in discriminating responses to "who is it" and "what is it" questions. The child was reinforced for placing the response cards on the appropriate color and learned the responses more efficiently this way. With another child, we constructed a peep-show window from a cardboard box in order to eliminate extraneous visual stimuli. We have also used gestures along with verbal stimuli. For example, when asking a "who" question, the clinician placed her hands directly in front of her. For a "what" question, her hands were out-stretched to the side. In this case, the child responded more appropriately to gestures, so we paired his strong responses to the gestured S^D with the verbal S^D. Then we used a fading procedure to remove the gestured S^D and soon he responded in the presence of the verbal S^D alone.

Sometimes, the use of the written word serves as an important component of the S^D, particularly for children whose response in the presence of visual stimuli is significantly better than it is in the presence of auditory stimuli. We have used the procedures described by Sulzbacher and Costello (1970) to teach Neil, whom we described earlier as having outstanding ability to read numbers and letters. We found that visual prompts assisted him in the acquisition of verbal skill. With another child, the use of a videotaped model resulted in an increase of appropriate language responses (Roth et al., 1972). Televised presentations have demonstrated reinforcing properties and their potential for the nonverbal child has not been adequately explored as yet.

MODIFYING SOCIAL INTERACTION

While clinicians are primarily concerned with verbal language, it is important that behavior which interferes with therapy be brought under control so that the child can be taught. Such behaviors as crying, biting, and head banging are disruptive in therapy and destructive to any social interaction. Zeilberger, Sampen, and Sloane (1968) reduced aggressive behavior in a four-and-a-half-year-old boy with a time out from positive reinforcement procedure. Bostow and Bailey (1969) describe a seven-year-old who was so destructive that he had to be tied to a door in a hallway because he could not be with other children. With reinforcement procedures, his aggressive behavior was virtually eliminated within a week, and he would even embrace other children. Kirby and Toler (1970) increased the interaction between an "isolate" boy and his classmates by having him pass out candy to them and providing reinforcement as soon as he completed the task. Schell and Adams (1968) directed parents to use conditioning procedures to produce desired changes in their child's behavior, and the results demonstrated improved social interaction.

At the clinic, we have observed verbal, physical, and object interactions with some of the children. Verbal interaction was defined as any verbal behavior, intelligible or not to the observer, involving another person. Physical interaction was defined as any physical contact between a child and another person. This did not include accidentally bumping into or falling on another person. Object interaction was defined as the manipulation of an object, not necessarily related to its appropriate use.

In our group program, Alan is now reported to be the most enthusiastic, most contacting and communicating of the children present. During his first semester in this group, out of 180 observations, his verbal interaction and physical interaction were zero, while his object interaction was 72%. The following semester his interaction pattern changed so that, of 180 observations, his verbal interaction was 31%, his physical interaction was 1%, and his object interaction was 52%. He became more eager to play and happy to be with other children.

When Neil entered our program he did not appear to recognize people, with the exception of his grandparents. He did not respond to people moving about, or to his parents' leaving the room. In addition to his individual therapy, he was placed into a group so that we could note the extent and quality of his social interaction. His behavior was observed at 10-second intervals for approximately 15-minute periods over three sessions. Out of a total of 217 observations, 179 or 71% were object interactions. There were no vocalizations or peer interactions. He did not respond to the clinician or the other children in the room.

In the training sessions, one of the procedures was to allow him to enter the room where a few clinicians were sitting around as if they were statues. They sat for 15 minutes, or until Neil recognized their presence by going over to one of them and touching, looking at, or saying something to her. For the first three sessions, he wandered about the room for the total time. During the fourth session, he interacted with the clinician after 12 minutes, at which time all of the clinicians cheered and clapped. It took less than one minute during the fifth session before he interacted. After the sixth session, he came directly into the room, went to a clinician and said, "Hi." As he learned their names, these were added, and a regular procedure was for him to say, "Hi, person," when he came into the room, and "Bye-bye, person," when he left. Now when Neil enters the center and sees one of the clinicians it is not unusual for him to run toward her with a smile, say, "Hi, person," and give her a hug and kiss.

We have attempted to observe interaction in a more systematic manner. We hope that we may determine the variables and manipulate one or more of them to effect more appropriate interaction. How do we increase social interaction? What conditions maximize the child's social interaction? What is the relationship of the child's language behavior to the physical environment and to the people in his presence? It is questions such as these to which we must address ourselves. The nonverbal child represents an enormous challenge for the clinician. The establishment of appropriate language behavior in a communicative context can be the result of a systematic, empirically based program. In this paper we have tried to highlight some of the problems, procedures, and new directions we must take.

APPENDIX Queens College Speech and Hearing Center

Child _____ Recorder _____ Date _____ Page _____

TRIAL	S^D	Pro	Mod	R	S^R	COMMENT

Summary: Trials:
S^D:
CORRECT R:

REFERENCES

Bloom, L., *Language Development: Form and Function in Emerging Grammars.* Cambridge, Mass.: MIT Press (1970).

Bloom, L., Why not pivot grammar? *J. Speech Hearing Dis., 36,* 40-51 (1971).

Bostow, D. E., and Bailey, J., Modification of severe disruptive and aggressive behavior using brief time out and reinforcement procedures. *J. Appl. Behav. Anal., 2,* 31-37 (1969).

Braine, M.D.S., The ontogeny of English phrase structure: The first phase. *Language, 39,* 1-13 (1963).

Bricker, W., and Bricker, D., A program of language training for the severely language handicapped child. *Except. Child, 37,* 101-111 (1970).

Brown, R., and Bellugi, U., Three processes in the child's acquisition of syntax. *Harv. Educ. Rev., 34,* 133-151 (1964).

Daly, D. A., Cantrell, R. P., Cantrell, M. L., and Aman, L. A., Structuring speech therapy contingencies with an oral apraxic child. *J. Speech Hearing Dis., 37,* 22-32 (1972).

Girardeau, F. L., and Spradlin, J. E., An introduction to the functional analysis of speech and language. In *A Functional Analysis Approach to Speech and Language: ASHA Monographs Number 14.* Washington, D.C.: American Speech and Hearing Association (January 1970).

Goldstein, S. B., and Lanyon, R. I., Parent-clinicians in the language training of an autistic child. *J. Speech Hearing Dis., 36,* 552-560 (1971).

Hartung, J. R., A review of procedures to increase verbal imitation skills and functional speech in autistic children. *J. Speech Hearing Dis., 35,* 203-217 (1970).

Kirby, F. D., and Toler, H. C., Modification of pre-school isolate behavior: A case study. *J. Appl. Behav. Anal., 3,* 309-314 (1970).

Leonard, L. B., A preliminary view of information theory and articulatory omissions. *J. Speech Hearing Dis., 36,* 511-517 (1971).

Lovaas, I., A program for the establishment of speech in psychotic children. In H. Sloane and B. MacAulay (Eds.), *Operant Procedures in Remedial Speech and Language Training.* Boston: Houghton Mifflin (1968).

McReynolds, L. V., and Huston, K., Token loss in speech imitation training. *J. Speech Hearing Dis., 36,* 486-495 (1971).

Miller, W., and Ervin, S., The development of grammar in child language. In U. Bellugi and R. Brown (Eds.), *The Acquisition of Language.* Monograph No. 29. Chicago: Society for Research in Child Development (1964).

Roth, F., Veth, E., Garrett, T., Rosembaum, R., and Wisan, A., The use of a video-taped model to expand language forms in an autistic child. Paper presented at the New York State Speech and Hearing Association, Ellenville, N.Y. (April 1972).

Ryan, B. P., Operant procedures applied to stuttering therapy for children. *J. Speech Hearing Dis., 36,* 264-281 (1971).

Schell, R. E., and Adams, W. P., Training parents of a young child with profound behavior deficits to be teacher therapists. *J. Spec. Educ., 2,* 439-455 (1968).

Shaw, C. K., and Shrum, W. F., The effects of response-contingent reward on the connected speech of children who stutter. *J. Speech Hearing Dis., 37,* 75-88 (1972).

Skinner, B. F., *Verbal Behavior.* New York: Appleton-Century-Crofts (1957).

Sulzbacher, S. I., and Costello, J. M., A behavioral strategy for language training of a child with autistic behaviors. *J. Speech Hearing Dis., 35,* 256-276 (1970).

Zeilberger, J., Sampen, S. E., and Sloane, H. N., Modification of a child's problem behaviors in the home with the mother as therapist. *J. Appl. Behav. Anal., 1,* 47-53 (1968).

A REVIEW OF PROCEDURES
TO INCREASE VERBAL IMITATION SKILLS
AND FUNCTIONAL SPEECH
IN AUTISTIC CHILDREN

Jurgen R. Hartung

A review of the substantial literature on the conditioning of verbal behavior in nonspeaking autistic children shows that a dearth of information and organized knowledge exists in this area of psychology. Although numerous separate articles have been published dealing with the effects of conditioning techniques on verbal behavior, only a few articles to date profess to present a systematic account of how to go about developing speech in nonspeaking children (Lovaas et al., 1966; Lovaas, 1968; MacAulay, 1968; Risley and Wolf, 1967; Sloane, Johnson, and Harris, 1968). The remaining studies focus primarily on the results of the authors' particular conditioning methods, give very limited or no rationale for the methods they use, and fail to base and support the progressive steps of their conditioning procedures on theoretical implications of verbal learning. Characteristically, these articles report the operant level of the three or so subjects used, describe the effectiveness of different reinforcers for each of the subjects, and give a rather limited perspective of the progress due to reinforcement (for example, one word in session I to 75 words in session XV). Worst of all, they provide the reader insufficient information about how they carried out their operant procedures.

Reprinted from *Journal of Speech and Hearing Disorders*, 1970, *35*, 203-217. Copyright 1970 by American Speech and Language Society. Reprinted by permission.

Jurgen R. Hartung is at the Mental Health Division, Department of Public Health and Welfare, County of San Mateo, California.

This paper was prepared under Rehabilitation Services Administration Training Grant Number 11-T-69 from the Social and Rehabilitation Service of the U.S. Department of Health, Education, and Welfare, while the author was a graduate student in clinical psychology. The author wishes to express his appreciation to Paul Dokecki of the University of Houston for his helpful suggestions and editorial comments.

This paper was written essentially as a reaction to such limitations in the literature concerning the verbal conditioning of nonspeaking children, primarily those whose condition is diagnosed as infantile autism. The objectives of the paper are threefold. First, an attempt is made to demonstrate the importance of establishing verbal behavior in nonspeaking autistic children. Second, some of the theoretical foundations underlying verbal conditioning are discussed. And finally, the procedures and related theoretical implications are reviewed in some detail.

Through this paper, I also hope to compensate for the lack of direction and guidance given to the reader in previous verbal conditioning reports. Instead of reviewing many different methods in toto, the important stages and trends of the verbal conditioning process are presented in a step-by-step fashion, incorporating the ideas and work of many contributors. The paper thus outlines a procedure by which speech may be established. What follows is a convenient, nonexhaustive list of suggestions, and some theoretical foundations, which have been useful to me and which may prove useful to others. It is important to keep in mind that the following procedures must be adapted to fit the needs of the individual child. A cookbook approach does not do justice to the child's level of functioning, nor does it recognize the sensitivity of operant work to individual variation.

THE VITAL IMPORTANCE OF SPEECH FOR RECOVERY

Experience with autistic children has disclosed that about half of all autistic children use speech, while the others are mute. For example, from a sample of 24 autistic children, Rimland (1964) found 10 who did not speak. These non-speaking children can be extremely poor prognostic risks. From follow-up studies, Kanner and Eisenberg (1955) found that the presence or absence of speech by age five has important prognostic implications. Almost without exception, those children who had not developed speech by the age of five failed to improve their level of socialization in later years. From a study of the autistic child in adolescence, Eisenberg (1956) showed the significant relationship of speech to recovery. He reported that of 32 children who had useful speech by the age of five, 16 obtained "fair" to "good" social adjustment, while only one out of 31 from the nonspeaking group reached the "fair" level. Early speech, then, seems to be an important factor. At the present state of our knowledge and experience, it is almost impossible to determine how useful speech must be before a child can make some degree of social adjustment. It is also unclear as to how socialized the child must be in order for speech to develop. Although speech sometimes can be developed via special procedures, this does not necessarily insure good social adjustment. What we do know is that the child who fails to use speech before the age of five is the one who makes the worst social adjustment and suffers the most in later years.

THE ROLE OF IMITATION IN FUNCTIONAL SPEECH

Although there remains a great deal of controversy over the role of imitation in speech, I believe that normal children initially acquire words by hearing speech. Perhaps it is not until the child has heard certain sounds over and over again that he will mimic these sounds as others produce them. During normal development, these verbal imitations probably are selectively reinforced in such a manner that a complex verbal repertoire develops. Having accepted this theory as a fundamentally correct view of verbal learning, Lovaas et al. (1966) claim that the first step in creating speech is to establish conditions in which imitation of vocal sounds will be learned. This implies that if a child is to learn to speak, it is necessary not only that he vocalize but also that his vocalizations be brought under the control of the vocal stimuli of others. Risley and Wolf (1967) went one step further by stating that the presence or absence of echolalia (a term applied primarily to autistic children who will consistently mimic the verbal productions of others) is an important predictor of ease of establishing more normal speech.

Clearly related, but more affirmative in nature, is the major theoretical assumption underlying the principles and methods presented here. Not only is imitative verbal behavior considered a prerequisite to functional speech, but functional speech cannot be developed in a nonspeaking child unless that child first imitates the verbal responses of others consistently. Once the child can imitate most words, phrases, and sentences, a diversified topography of verbal behavior can be produced by individual prompting. In accounting for the progress of an autistic child, Wolf, Risley, and Mees (1964) stated:

> Dicky's ability to mimic entire phrases and sentences was apparently crucial to the rapid progress in verbal training. . . without this mimicking behavior a long and arduous handshaping procedure would have been necessary to establish responses of the required topography. (p. 311)

THE FAILURE TO IMITATE

One of the most striking features of the autistic child's behavior is his apparent inability to imitate. While imitation is a prominent response disposition in normal young children, autistic children typically do not imitate other people. An exception, however, applies to those autistic children who rather spontaneously become echolalic usually at or beyond the age of six years.

No clear understanding prevails as to why children imitate or fail to imitate. Some writers (Piaget, 1951; Ritvo and Provence, 1953) seem to hold to the idea that a self-world kind of confusion is the basis for imitative behavior. Ritvo and Provence hypothesize that the child fails to imitate or imitates less because of a limited self, non-self differentiation. If this is the case, autistic children might profit from an increased emphasis on the exploration of boundaries and limits of their own bodies. One way of doing this is to select imitative responses to be learned that would enhance awareness of self, non-self differentiation (as in "pat-a-cake," "bye-bye" kissing, "so big," and the words "I" and "yes").*

The nonspeaking autistic child, then, characteristically fails to imitate the behavior of others before the age of five. As a result, he never passes through what appears to be a necessary stage in speech development and thus ends up not using speech by the time he is five years old. This child has a very poor chance of making any sort of "normal" social adjustment.

STAGES AND TRENDS IN CONDITIONING VERBAL REPERTOIRES

The Training Environment

The training environment may vary depending upon the particular stage of conditioning or the needs of the child at the time. At the onset, a room with limited possibilities for distractions is recommended (that is, simple furniture, nonbreakables). Such a setting will usually lower the occurrence of disruptive behavior. One researcher (Hewett, 1965) developed a special isolation booth which, because of its limited size, made disruptive behavior almost impossible. The booth was divided into sections by a shutter which the clinician could raise and lower. The section for the child contained a chair facing the shutter which, when raised, revealed the section where the clinician sat facing the subject. A light focused on the clinician's side of the booth. When the shutter was lowered, the subject was deprived of light, rewards, and the presence of the clinician.

The Limitation of Disruptive Behavior

The limitation of disruptive behavior becomes particularly important when working with nonspeaking autistic children, who in general tend to be quite disruptive and destructive in their behavior. Some ways of limiting such

---

*Autistic children almost never use the words "I" and "yes" until they are six or seven years old, or until echolalia occurs.

behavior are suggested here. One simple method allows the clinician to physically restrain a child by holding the child's legs between his legs while working on verbal behavior.

Lovaas et al. (1966) found a more direct approach to be quite successful. He delivered punishment (spanking and shouting by an adult) for inattentive, self-destructive, and tantrumous behavior which interfered with the training. Most of the undesirable behaviors were thereby suppressed within one week. Incorrect vocal behavior was never punished and should never be punished.

Risley and Wolf (1967) use a technique which they call "time-out from positive reinforcement." When mild disruptive behavior occurs, the clinician merely looks away from the child. For highly disruptive behavior, the time-out procedure involves both extinction of the behavior and removal of the reinforcer—the clinician either leaves the room with the reinforcer or the child is removed to an isolated room.

These procedures should not be tried out haphazardly on a particular child. The method chosen should be geared to the child's needs and be used consistently until the child's behavior requires a different approach. An exception, however, applies to general methods of restraint. A clinician may hold the child's legs in his own or in some other manner physically restrict the child's movements while still effectively applying one of the other techniques mentioned.

Conditioning Attention and Eye Contact

Before operant procedures can be utilized satisfactorily, the clinician must have the attention of his subject. Since nonspeaking autistic children are characterized by an unusually limited span of attention, as well as an almost complete failure to attend to other people in general, it is imperative that the clinician first establish some control over this behavior. Imitative behavior appears to be partly contingent upon eye contact and other-directed attention. The child who does not attend adequately to outside cues is incapable of modifying his behavior accordingly and will hardly establish an imitative repertoire leading to the effective use of language.

Risley et al. (1967) maintain the child's attention by having the clinician hold the reinforcer directly in front of his own face. Since the child will tend to look at the reinforcer (in this case food), this procedure ensures that he will be looking toward the clinician's face.

The use of loud noises and manual guidance are more direct and sometimes more effective ways of drawing the child's attention. Slapping a table top loudly or slapping the child's knee seems to draw immediate attention. Yelling or shouting the child's name or some appropriate phrase is also effective. Sometimes the clinician may find it beneficial to yell the word or phrase to be learned. Finally, holding or turning the child's head so that he faces the clinician may be useful.

Blake and Moss (1967), using Hewett's isolation booth, shaped eye contact by first leaving the subject in total darkness. Then, every five seconds, the clinician opened the shutter, put on the lights, and said, "Hi, Dolly, look at me!" Rewards were made contingent on the subject's looking in the direction of the clinician. If the subject looked elsewhere, the shutter was dropped for 15 seconds.

The Transition from Motor to Verbal Imitative Behavior

In reference to the training of autistic children, Goldstein (1959) has said:

These children learn only by doing: through specific movements and activities, they can be brought into contact with a desired task. (p. 549)

Experience with autistic children has shown that, to a large extent, Goldstein seems to be right. For instance, autistic children do appear to learn motor imitations more readily than verbal imitations, especially at the beginning of an operant conditioning program. From such evidence, I would argue in favor of conditioning a repertoire of consistent motor imitative behaviors before actually beginning vocal training.

For a detailed account of conditioning motor imitative behavior, the reader is referred to Baer, Peterson, and Sherman (1967) and Peterson (1968). Only the transition from motor to verbal imitative behavior will be described here.

When the subject reaches the level where he imitates almost every new motor performance, vocal training is begun. The clinician now says, "Do this" ("Do this" is used to precede all motor and verbal imitative examples); but instead of making a motor response, he makes a vocal response. If the subject then fails to imitate the vocal response, the vocal response is set into a chain of nonvocal responses, progressively fading out the motor response component.

For example, the clinician might say, "Do this," rise from his chair and walk to the center of the room, turn towards the subject, say a word or syllable, and return to his seat. Such coupling of motor and vocal responses may be maintained for several demonstrations during which time the motor performance is made successively shorter and more economical of motion until finally the clinician can remain in his seat and elicit imitative verbal responses from the subject.

A study by Risley (1968) demonstrates this use of imitative skills to develop complex performances. Risley developed the children's ability to imitate by starting with gross motor imitations, progressing to fine motor imitations, then to facial responses, and at the end added verbalizations. He defined a "complex performance" as the child's ability to perform the four acts simultaneously. As an example, a child might be expected to have his arms out to the side, palms of his hands turned back, face frowning, and make the statement, "This too shall pass away." The ultimate and successfully completed intent of this type of imitation training was to give the children the ability to listen to novel language performances and to repeat them.

The Systematic Selection of Vocal Responses

Lovaas et al. (1966) list three useful criteria for selecting vocal sounds that the nonspeaking child may readily learn:

1. Vocal sounds may be selected that can be prompted by manually moving the child through the sound. For instance, the clinician might emit the sound /b/, holding the child's lips closed with his fingers and quickly removing them when the child exhales.

2. The second criterion for the selection of words or sounds centers on their concomitant visual components. Such sounds as those of the labial consonant /m/ and front vowels such as /a/ are examples. In each case, the clinician should exaggerate their articulation.

3. Those words or sounds that the child already can use (those most frequently used) may be selected for training.

Lovaas et al. (1966) found that children would discriminate words with visual components more easily than those with only auditory components (the consonants /k/, /g/, /s/, and /l/ were very difficult for the nonspeaking autistic child and were mastered later than other sounds).

Establishing Control Over Vocal Responses

The assumption that children learn to speak by first imitating the vocal responses of others makes this, then, the most crucial stage in verbal conditioning. The procedure described here comes mainly from the work of Lovaas et al. (1966) with nonspeaking emotionally disturbed children, although the ideas of various other contributors are also included.

Initially, the child should be rewarded for all vocalizations and for visually fixating on the adult's mouth and/or eyes. Even those vocalizations that at first appear meaningless in terms of affecting later verbal behavior should be rewarded. Blake and Moss (1967) demonstrated the significance of reinforcing just such a general type of vocalization. They put a crying child into Hewett's (1965) isolation booth. The child learned that when she stopped crying, pretty colors being presented on a screen would go off. At first the child deliberately cried to reinstate the colors, but slowly the crying shifted to babbling sounds.

The child may now be rewarded only if he emits a sound within the prescribed time after an adult has emitted a sound. Some clinicians favor emitting a sound or word every 10 seconds, while others present words more frequently, on the order of one about every four to five seconds. The time allotted for the child to respond is also somewhat arbitrary, although some investigators have followed the policy of progressively shortening the interval between the clinician's vocalization and the child's vocalizations as training proceeds.

The next stage requires that the child be rewarded only if the sound he emitted within the prescribed time interval resembled the adult's sound. Most children will require prompting to complete this stage. By holding and guiding the child's lips, the clinician usually can evoke the desired response. The prompting is then gradually faded, first by moving the fingers away from the mouth to the cheek, then by placing them gently on the jaw, and finally by removing them from the child's face altogether. Now the child should be able to reproduce the response without any further prompting. Finally, the child is rewarded only if his vocalizations very closely match the clinician's vocalizations—that is, if the child's response was imitative.

Once the child reliably and immediately imitates his first word, a new word may be presented. The two words should then be presented alternately. New words should always be interspersed with old words, since a new response has not been learned (added to the child's vocabulary) until the child can reproduce the word when it is presented again after other words have been learned, and following a passage of time.

The Sudden Emergence of Echolalia

After the child acquires the first word, the clinician may encounter a great deal of resistance from the child before the second word is learned. The child essentially resists by taking a great deal more time to imitate the second word than he did the first word. Although such a manner of responding appears to be characteristic at this level of verbal training, it also seems directly related to a rather unsuspected occurrence—the sudden emergence of echolalia. To quote from Risley and Wolf (1967):

> Usually by the second or third word, a general imitative response class will have been established, i.e., the child will then reliably and immediately imitate any new word. (p. 77)

A number of investigators have observed and described this phenomenon in their own studies, but have failed to notice that this pattern also occurs somewhat consistently in other studies. For example, Hewett (1965) reported:

> Once the first two words "go" and "my" were learned, Peter's speech became echolalic and he readily attempted to imitate all words the teachers said. (p. 933)

A study by Isaacs, Thomas, and Goldiamond (1960) reveals that a form of "sudden echolalia" also seems to occur among previously nonspeaking adult schizophrenics:

> At the sixth session (at the end of week six), when the experimenter said, "Say gum, gum," the subject suddenly said, "Gum please." This response was accompanied by reinstatement of other responses of this class, that is, the subject answered questions regarding his name and age. Thereafter, he responded to questions by the experimenter both in individual sessions and in group sessions, but answered to no one else. (p. 9).

I first observed this phenomenon in the very early stages of a program designed to condition verbal behavior in a nonspeaking autistic boy. Following the accurate and reliable imitation of the word "please," the subject refused to imitate another word for two full months, even under the pressure of excessive prodding. At the end of the two-month period, he finally mimicked the words "potato chip." Two more weeks were required before he could successfully combine the words "please" and "potato chip" to form the request "please potato chip." Once this was accomplished, the subject suddenly began to echo almost every word and some short phrases. Generally, all one-syllable words were clearly imitated. Words of two or more syllables were more often imitated crudely, if at all. At first the subject only imitated me, but eventually his imitative response generalized somewhat to other adults. Although he generalized a few words to many people, he continued to reliably and immediately imitate only me.

Perhaps by becoming suddenly echolalic, the child is expressing a change in his feelings for a particular adult. The initial resistance to communication, the sudden appearance of echolalia, and the tendency to imitate only that one person who has been the supplier of rewards suggest that the autistic child has stepped out of his encapsulated world to allow himself momentarily to relate to and feel affection for another person.

The Phenomenon of Silent Speech

A number of equally valid explanations can be given to account for the sudden emergency of echolalia. Possibly, the autistic child possessed an inner vocabulary all along which he failed to express until he became echolalic. Such an explanation could account for the sudden acquisition and unusually good pronunciation of words characteristic of the echolalic stage. A closer inspection of the speech characteristics of autistic children suggests that this is a reasonable interpretation.

The speech patterns of autistic children seem to indicate that many of these children develop an unexpressed side of speech but fail to develop the expressive side. A good example of this is the fact that whispering seems to be common among nonspeaking autistic children. The whispering however, is almost always noncommunicative and unintelligible. The autistic child may initially acquire words silently by hearing them, and it is not until he is willing to imitate the vocalizations of others that his range of words becomes apparent.

Lending further support to this theory is the observation that frequently those autistic children who do not speak are the very ones who had an unusually advanced vocabulary when they were younger. Wolff and Chess (1965) feel that the unusual use of metaphor and symbolic language characteristic of both the speaking and the nonspeaking autistic child appears to be the outcome of a relatively advanced level of language development distorted by "repetitive clinging to former modes of expression. . . ."

That nonspeaking autistic children possess a silent vocabulary was demonstrated by an autistic child known to me. All those persons in close daily contact with the child, such as his parents, his teachers, and his clinician, reported having heard his occasional whispering, which they were, however, only infrequently able to understand because of the low volume and idiosyncratic words. The child also displayed unusually good pronunciation once echolalia began. He was able to pronounce well such difficult words as "San Francisco" after just one attempt. Soon after echolalia became a prominent feature of the boy's verbal behavior, I found he could count from one to 10. The clarity and rapidity with which he could do this supports the belief that an inner, unexpressed speech facility must have been in existence for some time.

The Transition from Imitation to Naming

The following is an integration of the procedures used by Risley and Wolf (1967), Lovaas et al. (1966), and me. Naming is defined as the emission of an appropriate verbal response in the presence of some stimulus object. After imitative responses occur with high probability and short latency following each verbal prompting, stimulus control is shifted from the verbal promptings (imitation) to appropriate objects and pictures (naming).

A picture or object is presented with the verbal prompting, and the child is reinforced for imitating the name. Then the imitative prompting is faded out while the child continues to receive reinforcement for saying the name of the object: (1) the clinician holds up an object (with the reinforcer behind the object) and asks, "What is this?" When the child looks at it, the clinician immediately prompts with the object's name. The child is reinforced for imitating the prompting. When the child is reliably looking at the object without the food being held behind it, the time between the question "What is this?" and the prompting is gradually lengthened to more than five seconds. If after several trials the child continues to wait for the presentation of the verbal prompting, partial prompting is given, for example, "trr" for train. If the correct response does not occur within about three seconds more, the complete prompting is then presented. A correct response results in a bite of food and a social reward such as "right" or "good." (2) When the child begins saying the name when only the partial prompting is presented, the clinician continues the above procedure but begins to say the partial prompting more softly. (3) Whenever the child inappropriately imitates the question "What is this?" a time-out is programmed, that is, the object is withdrawn and the clinician looks down at the table, maintaining about 10 seconds of silence.

Answering Questions

Two methods of fading out prompting stimuli are suggested for teaching the child to answer questions. The first method is similar to that used to establish naming. (1) First, teach the child to imitate "How are you? Fine." Then the question is faded by gradually lengthening the time between the question, "How are you?" and the answer, "Fine," to more than five seconds. This procedure does not involve fading in the usually applied sense of that word (as in method 2). One advantage of lengthening the time interval between the stimulus question, "How are you?" and the response, "Fine!" is that many children will tend to give an anticipatory response, saying, "Fine" before the clinician prompts that response. Thus, by lengthening the interval between question and answer, the clinician is establishing proper stimulus control of new responses. (2) The child first is given both the question and answer ("How are you? Fine.") for imitation. Gradually the question part is faded by saying it softly and quickly while emphasizing the answer ("How are you? FINE.").*

The Establishment of Phrases

The first step in establishing phrases is the same as the procedure used to teach individual words: (1) Mimicking of phrases is reinforced until the phrases are consistently imitated. (2) Then control should be shifted to appropriate circumstances by introducing partial promptings (the first word or two of a phrase), which are gradually faded out. Sentences such as "that's a _____"

---

*This method also can be used effectively to establish "naming" (for example, "What is this? DOG!").

or "I want _____" may be taught using vocabulary words that the child already knows. (3) Finally, more varied sentences such as "My name is _____," "I live at _____," or "I am _____ years old" can be taught.

Conditioning Functional Speech

At this point in verbal training, social and natural reinforcers can be used to maintain the variety of phrases learned. If the child can be shown that his verbal responses change something in his immediate environment, leading to a personal satisfaction, then it is more probable that language will become spontaneous and situationally appropriate. The socially rewarding value of an appropriate response may be taught the child in the following way: The clinician says, "Open the door," when the child wants out. If the child imitates the sentence, the clinician opens the door. Next, the partial prompting "Open" is used for the same procedure. This partial prompting is gradually faded out until the clinician can put his hand on the doorknob, look at the child, and expect the child to respond with, "Open the door." The latter promptings of a hand on the doorknob and looking are also faded out and replaced with, "What do you want?" This is done by mumbling the question softly as the child and clinician approach the door and then increasing the volume on succeeding trials. Whenever the child inappropriately imitates "What do you want?" the clinician should repeat the question at a lower volume and follow it with a loud partial prompt (for example, "What do you want? OPEN"). On succeeding trials the partial prompting, "Open," is then decreased in volume until the child responds to the closed door and question with, "Open the door."

The particular likes and dislikes of a child may serve as effective natural reinforcers. For one autistic boy, having a hand placed on the top of his head was aversive. His immediate reaction was to squirm away. The clinician made use of this by placing his hand firmly atop the child's head and simultaneously saying "Stop it." The child, being echolalic, immediately responded with "Stop it," at which point the clinician quickly removed his hand. Within 30 minutes, the child no longer needed the clinician's prompt to respond correctly with "Stop it" each time a hand was placed on his head. (The statement "Stop it" occurred spontaneously on one of the trials; fading was not required.) A week passed before the clinician again placed his hand on the child's head. Without prompting, the child immediately shouted, "Stop it!" Elaborations of the phrase were subsequently introduced by adding more words (for example, "Stop it, Jurgen. Please stop it, Jurgen").

The Generalization of Appropriate Speech

Newly acquired appropriate speech often will spontaneously generalize to situations outside the specific conditioning environment. Self-initiated speech seems to generalize primarily because of its functional value for the child—the child soon discovers that by using words he can more effectively satisfy his desires. The reason imitative verbal behavior generalizes is much less obvious. Baer, Peterson, and Sherman (1967) suggest that imitative behavior eventually develops reinforcing properties of its own. Because the child is consistently rewarded for responding like the adult, the concept of similarity becomes associated with food, and similarity becomes a secondary reinforcer. Thus, a child can provide himself with rewards by imitating adult behavior. Once established, verbal imitations may be maintained by periodic adult reinforcement.

These explanations may account for the generalization of verbal behavior in both normal and abnormal children. However, newly acquired words do not spontaneously generalize as readily in nonspeaking emotionally disturbed children as they do in normal children. It is therefore recommended that the clinician extend generalization systematically. This can be accomplished in a number of ways:

1. Reinforce appropriate speech in a variety of situations such as in the home, in a car, in stores, or out of doors in settings familiar and interesting to the child.

2. Train the child to respond to a variety of individuals. Family members, caretakers, and even other children may be used as reinforcing agents. Strait (1958) found that generalization was facilitated by gradually bringing other people into the therapy room. It may be particularly beneficial to have the child's parents administer the reinforcers during occasional sessions.

3. Select words for training that have relevance to the child (for example, "cookie" instead of "zebra" or "I am very tired" instead of "This too shall pass").

4. Make optimal use of social and natural reinforcers. For example, with the correct response, the clinician should immediately say "Good" or "That's right." Such a verbal statement, besides bridging the gap between the appropriate response and the presentation of the food (making reinforcement contingencies more precise), also favors generalization to verbal reinforcers (social reinforcers). Probably the most effective way to take advantage of naturally occurring events is to train the parents or other caretakers in the use of the operant procedures being applied.

The reader is again reminded that these procedures should not be taken as fixed and unchanging. One of the advantages of a behavioral technique lies in the possibilities of refining its procedures and adapting them to specific human problems.

Imitation as a Precursor of Identification

The significance of imitation as a precursor to functional speech has been emphasized in this paper in two related ways. First of all, some evidence was presented to demonstrate that verbal imitative behavior appears to precede the development of more complex verbal behavior. Secondly, it was shown that an imitative repertoire is a prerequisite for each of the major stages of verbal conditioning. The successful implementation of verbal training thus assumes that the child already imitates the verbal responses of others consistently.

A deeper analysis of imitative behavior reveals that imitation may also be the precursor of some other behavioral attribute. The observation that the child does not imitate indiscriminately (those he likes he imitates the most) suggests the imitation may be related in some manner to identification.

Church (1961) believes that the social significance of imitative responses resides largely in their capacity for fostering adult-child interactions. He points out:

> Imitation early becomes a vehicle of playful communication between child and adult. . . . Moreover, the infant's imitative responses may prolong adult-child interactions and thus facilitate the development of attachment behavior. (p. 34)

The sudden emergence of echolalia may be a direct expression of such "attachment" behavior in previously nonspeaking autistic children. Possibly echolalia is the first concrete sign that some degree of identification has occurred between the child and his clinician. In this respect, one may be justified in concluding that, by conditioning an imitative verbal repertoire, the clinician is essentially fostering the process of identification. Bandura (1965) explains this process in terms of Mowrer's (1950, 1960) reinforcement theory of identification:

> The secondary reinforcement theory of identification assumes that as a model mediates rewards for a child, the model's behavioral attributes acquire secondary reinforcing properties through the process of classical conditioning. On the basis of stimulus generalization, matching responses attain rewarding value for the child in proportion to their similarity to those exhibited by the model. Consequently, the child can administer conditioned reinforcers to himself simply by reproducing as closely as possible the model's positively valenced behavior. The theory would predict, therefore, that the condition in which children received direct positive reinforcement would produce the greatest amount of imitation, with the model who dispensed the rewards serving as the main source of behavior. (p. 338)

Identification, then, may in a sense be considered a deferred and more comprehensive form of imitation. Perhaps in the process of identification we may find the real key to functional speech.

REFERENCES

Baer, D., Peterson, R., and Sherman, J., The development of imitation by reinforcing behavioral similarity as a model. *J. Exp. Anal. Behav., 10,* 405-416 (1967).

Bandura, A., Behavioral modification through modeling procedures. In L. Krasner and L. Ullman (Eds.), *Research in Behavior Modification.* New York: Holt, Rinehart and Winston (1965).

Blake, P., and Moss, T., The development of socialization skills in an electively mute child. *Behav. Res. Ther., 5,* 349-356 (1967).

Church, J., *Language and the Discovery of Reality: A Developmental Psychology of Cognition.* New York: Random House (1961).

Eisenberg, L., The autistic child in adolescence. *Amer. J. Psychiat., 112,* 607-612 (1956).

Goldstein, K., Abnormal mental conditions in infancy. *J. Nerv. Ment. Dis., 48,* 538-557 (1959).

Hewett, F., Teaching speech in an autistic child through operant conditioning. *Amer. J. Orthopsychiat., 35,* 927-936 (1965).

Isaacs, W., Thomas, J., and Goldiamond, I., Application of operant conditioning to reinstate verbal behavior in psychotics. *J. Speech Hearing Dis., 25,* 8-12 (1960).

Kanner, L., and Eisenberg, L., Notes on the follow-up studies of autistic children. In P. Hoch and J. Zubin (Eds.), *Psychopathology of Childhood.* New York: Grune and Stratton (1955).

Lovaas, I., Berberich, J., Perloff, B., and Schaeffer, B., Acquisition of imitative speech by schizophrenic children. *Science, 151,* 705-707 (1966).

Lovaas, I., A program for the establishment of speech in psychotic children. In H. Sloane and B. MacAulay (Eds.), *Operant Procedures in Remedial Speech and Language Training.* Boston: Houghton Mifflin (1968).

MacAulay, B., A program for teaching speech and beginning reading to non-verbal retardates. In H. Sloane and B. MacAulay (Eds.), *Operant Procedures in Remedial Speech and Language Training.* Boston: Houghton Mifflin (1968).

Mowrer, O., Identification: A link between learning theory and psychotherapy. In O. Mowrer, *Learning Theory and Personality Dynamics.* New York: Ronald (1950).

Mowrer, O., *Learning Theory and the Symbolic Process.* New York: Wiley (1960).

Peterson, R., Imitation: A basic behavioral mechanism. In H. Sloane and B. MacAulay (Eds.), *Operant Procedures in Remedial Speech and Language Training.* Boston: Houghton Mifflin (1968).

Piaget, J., *Play, Dreams and Imitation in Childhood.* New York: W. W. Norton (1951), pp. 73-74.

Rimland, B., *Infantile Autism.* New York: Appleton-Century-Crofts (1964).

Risley, T., and Wolf, M., Establishing functional speech in echolalic children. *Behav. Res. Ther., 5,* 73-88 (1967).

Risley, T., Learning and lollipops. *Psychol. Today* (January, 1968).

Ritvo, S., and Provence, S., Form perception and imitation in some autistic children: Diagnostic findings and their contextual interpretation. *Psychoanal. Stud. Child, 8,* 155-161 (1953).

Sloane, H., Johnson, M., and Harris, F., Remedial procedures for teaching verbal behavior to speech deficient or defective young children. In H. Sloane and B. MacAulay (Eds.), *Operant Procedures in Remedial Speech and Language Training.* Boston: Houghton Mifflin (1968).

Strait, R., A child who was speechless in school and social life. *J. Speech Hearing Dis., 23,* 253-254 (1958).

Wolf, M., Risley, T., and Mees, H., Application of operant conditioning procedures to the behavior problems of an autistic child. *Behav. Res. Ther., 1,* 305-312 (1964).

Wolff, S., and Chess, S., An analysis of the language of fourteen schizophrenic children. *J. Child Psychol. Psychiat., 6,* 29-41 (1965).

A RAPID METHOD
OF ELIMINATING STUTTERING
BY A REGULATED BREATHING APPROACH

N. H. Azrin
R. G. Nunn

Summary—The Habit Reversal Procedure for eliminating nervous habits was applied to the problem of stuttering. In the new procedure the speaker interrupted his speech at moments of actual or anticipated stuttering and at natural pause points, and resumed speaking immediately after breathing deeply during the pause. In addition to this regularized pausing and breathing, the program included other factors such as formulation of one's thoughts prior to speaking, identification of stutter-prone situations, identification of mannerisms associated with stuttering, speaking for short durations when tense or nervous, daily breathing exercises, relaxation procedures for anxiety, immediate display of improved speaking, and enlisting family support for progress. Fourteen stutterers were given training in the program during a single counseling session of about two hours duration. The next day, the average number of stuttering episodes decreased by 94 per cent, by 97 per cent at the end of one month, and by 99 per cent during the extended follow-up. Each of the clients was improved by at least 93 per cent. The new procedure appears to be more rapid and effective than alternative procedures.

Stuttering is a problem about which much is known from laboratory studies, but for which no generally effective treatment has been developed as also has been concluded in a recent review by Ingham and Andrews (1973). Beech

Reprinted from *Behavior Research and Therapy*, 1974, *12*, 279-286. Copyright 1974 by Pergamon Press, Inc. Reprinted by permission.

N. H. Azrin and R. G. Nunn are both at the Behavior Research Laboratory, Anna State Hospital, Anna, Illinois.

and Fransella (1968) similarly concluded from their review of stuttering research that "No single or multiple form of treatment is characterized by more than a modest degree of success" (p. 15).

Perhaps the most effective method of eliminating stuttering in laboratory situations is the "rhythm" or "metronome" procedure in which the stutterer speaks in time with a regular beat (Barber, 1940; Jones and Azrin, 1969; Fransella, 1967; Beech and Fransella, 1968; Azrin et al., 1968). Stuttering generally is reduced by about 90 per cent or more by that procedure in the laboratory. Jones and Azrin (1969) extended the utility of the procedure by having the stutterers speak several words between beats, interrupting the speech prior to each beat and resuming the speech again at each beat. When the rhythmic beat occurred about once every three seconds, the stutterers were able to speak fluently when they initiated speech at each beat and paused shortly before the next beat. The speech was found to sound natural to observers in contrast with the unnatural sound of speech that has been synchronized in a staccato fashion to more closely spaced beats. Goldiamond (personal communication) has described a procedure that has some similarity to the Jones and Azrin method. Goldiamond taught the stutterer to pause at natural stop points in his speech such as at the end of a phrase or clause, and has found his "juncturing" technique to be effective as well as yielding a natural sounding speech pattern.

Stuttering may be considered from a different perspective: not as a specific speech problem but as one type of nervous habit. If considered as a type of nervous habit, the recently developed "Habit Reversal" procedure for the elimination of nervous habits might be useful. Azrin and Nunn (1973) developed this Habit Reversal Procedure to eliminate such diverse non-verbal nervous habits as fingernail-biting, thumb-sucking, hair-pulling, head-shaking, and one verbal habit, lisping. In general, the training program increased awareness of the habit and of habit-associated behaviors, identified habit-prone situations, displayed improvements conspicuously, and enlisted the social support of family and friends for self-control efforts. A central feature of the treatment was the use of a postural activity that was incompatible with the habit. This incompatible activity differed for each type of tic or habit. The client was taught to use this incompatible activity as a corrective reaction to stop the habit movement when the habit occurred and as a preventive reaction in habit-prone situations.

If this Habit-Reversal rationale were to be applied to stuttering, an incompatible activity to stuttering must be available. Here, the findings of Jones and Azrin (1969), and Goldiamond offer a possible solution in that the forced pausing in speech is known to inhibit stuttering in laboratory settings and might serve as the necessary incompatible activity to stuttering. In our preliminary efforts, however, simple pausing was not found to be sufficient.

Other features, therefore, were added, such as changes in the breathing pattern, self-induced relaxation and the formulation of one's thoughts. Beech and Fransella (1968) have summarized the several studies that have indicated the association of stuttering and irregularity of breathing.

The objective was to develop a procedure that would eliminate stuttering in the client's everyday life, would be effective for all clients, would be effective immediately, would require a minimum duration of counseling and would produce benefits that endured.

METHOD

The clients were 14 stutterers who responded to a newspaper advertisement offering treatment for nervous habits. As shown in Table 6.1, nine were male and five were female: their ages ranged from 4-67 yr (average of 38 yr). They had stuttered for an average of 24 yr (range: 2-65 yr). All 14 (except for the 4-yr old child) had received unsuccessful professional treatment for stuttering, usually from two or more therapists. At the start of the counseling session, they avoided speaking, especially those words on which they were likely to stutter and they reported doing the same in their everyday social interaction. The average number of times they stuttered was reported by them to be about three hundred per day.

All of them stuttered repeatedly during the counseling, two of them on almost every word, except for one who stuttered primarily on her name, and the other who stuttered primarily on words beginning with the letter M. All clients were accepted for treatment except for one who would not cooperate in the practice exercises during the counseling session and one client who was receiving disability welfare payments because of his stuttering and would not attempt to control his stuttering outside of the office.

All of the counseling was given in a single session of about 2 hr duration. No additional counseling sessions were given.

The specific procedures and their purposes are described only briefly below since they are identical to the procedures described in detail elsewhere in the Habit Reversal program for nervous habits (Azrin and Nunn, 1973). A lengthy description is given for the competing reaction to stuttering since the competing reaction selected for a given habit is distinctive to that habit.

Inconvenience Review

The client reviews the inconveniences and annoyances that have resulted from stuttering. This procedure heightens his motivation to engage in the necessary training effort.

TABLE 6.1. Individual stuttering frequencies of 14 clients before and after treatment

Client			Pre-treatment frequency of stuttering (per day)	One-month post-treatment frequency of stuttering (per day)	Number of words stuttered on telephone follow-up
Age (years)	Sex	Number of years stuttered			
25	female	12	10	0	0
37	female	23	45	0	0
23	male	17	30	0	0
44	female	34	500	8	0
25	female	17	2	0	0
44	male	36	10	2	0
30	male	27	1000	4	0
37	male	34	100	7	0
67	male	65	250	7	5
64	male	24	20	0	0
4	male	2	1000	0	0
19	male	15	100	4	0
9	female	6	150	0	0
26	male	23	1000	0	0
Mean $\bar{x} = 24$			$\bar{x} = 372$/day	$\bar{x} = 2$/day	$\bar{x} = 04$

Awareness Training

The client deliberately stutters and is required to describe in great detail the nature of the episode including the type of words stuttered, the situations or persons which provoke stuttering, and associated body movements such as eyeblinking or facial or hand-movements. This procedure clearly identifies for the client the circumstances under which he stutters so that he can prepare himself better for these circumstances. The procedure also teaches the client to focus his attention on each stuttering episode so he will be prepared to take action on every such episode.

Anticipation Awareness

The client is taught to alert himself to the likelihood of a stuttering episode. Whenever he feels as if he will stutter, he indicates this to the counselor by pausing in his speech. Also, the counselor alerts the client when he detects such stuttering-related signs as neck tensing, eyeblinking or hand-movements.

Relaxation Training

Several procedures are used to teach the client to relax himself when he becomes tense since tension is generally associated with stuttering. (1) In the Relaxed Posture Procedure, the client learns to sit and stand in comfortable postures by letting his shoulders drop slightly from their normal posture position and by slouching slightly, if necessary, since such postures tend to relax the muscles of the abdomen and chest which are usually tense when stuttering occurs. (2) In the Relaxed Breathing Procedure, he learns to breathe deeply, slowly and regularly since such breathing is relaxing and is opposite to the shallow, fast, irregular breathing associated with anxiety and stuttering. Specifically, he learns to inhale and exhale for an equal duration and without pausing at the upper or lower limits of the breathing cycle. (3) In the Self-Directed Relaxation Procedure, the client learns to facilitate his relaxation by telling himself to "Relax" while letting his abdominal and throat muscles go completely limp as he continues his Relaxed Breathing exercises.

Incompatible Activities

Stuttering requires speaking. One obvious incompatible reaction to stuttering is to discontinue speaking. Similarly, speaking requires exhalation of air and inhalation is incompatible with speaking. Several other factors seemed to be associated with not stuttering while speaking. If the client had mentally formulated his words before speaking, he seemed to stutter far less, perhaps because he need not falter for words. If he spoke for a short duration and paused as in the juncturing and rhythm procedure, he stuttered far less. If he took a deep breath before speaking, he seemed to stutter less when he resumed speaking. If he started his speech immediately after inhaling without holding his breath prior to speaking, he stuttered far less, perhaps because of the more relaxed state of the vocal musculature. This deep breathing also seemed to produce relaxation in opposition to the shallow rapid breathing associated with nervousness and anxiety (Jacobson, 1938). If he emphasized the first few syllables or words of his statement by changing the intensity or tone of his voice, he stuttered less, perhaps because of the partial "rhythm" thereby imparted to the speech. Taking all of these considerations into account, the competing activities to stuttering were to stop speaking, to take a deep breath by exhaling and then slowly inhaling, to consciously relax one's chest and throat muscles, to formulate mentally the words to be spoken, to start speaking immediately after taking a deep breath, to emphasize the initial part of a statement, and to speak for short durations. As the speech became more fluent, he gradually increased the duration of speech.

Corrective Training

The client was given practice in initiating the competing activities the instant he started stuttering. The counselor reminded him to stop speaking and to carry out the competing activities if the client failed to do so.

Preventive Training

The client was given practice in engaging in the competing activities when he anticipated that he would stutter. Also, when the counselor detected stuttering-associated mannerisms, or speech hesitancy, he signalled to the client to perform the competing activities.

Symbolic Rehearsal

The client imagined himself in stuttering prone situations and demonstrated, as well as described to the counselor the prescribed activities he would engage in within such circumstances.

Positive Practice

Several types of structured practice were given: (1) The client practiced the competing breathing pattern while reading, the number of words spoken per breath being progressively increased as he was able to speak more fluently. The client read the first line of a book while interrupting and breathing after each word. On the second line, he interrupted only after two words, on the third line after every third word, and so on until he was reading long phrases before pausing for a breath. If he faltered in his speech, he read one less word per breath on the next line, resuming the progressive increase in words-per-breath as soon as possible. (This deep breathing usually caused temporary drowsiness in the form of occasional yawnings.) (2) As he spoke to the counselor, he practiced the interrupt-and-breathe pattern. (3) While not speaking, he practiced the several Relaxation exercises. (4) All of the clients, except for the two children had major difficulty talking on a telephone. They were asked to telephone friends each day for the first few weeks to practice their new method of breathing and speaking on the phone. (5) A Telephone Group was established in which earlier clients telephoned the more recent clients. The two children were not included in this group. During their phone conversation, the more experienced clients offered encouragement to the more recent clients and answered questions they had about the procedures. For one client, telephone-call role-playing was used during the counseling session. (6) Additional speaking practice was given to the clients who had difficulty with specific letters or words. Using a dictionary they selected stuttering-prone words and practiced speaking whole sentences with these difficult words placed in different locations (beginning, middle and end) in the sentence.

Social Support

The client contacted interested friends or family members and told them of his progress and asked them to remind him to practice his new manner of breathing and speaking should they ever notice him beginning to stutter. In the case of the two small children, they described the procedures to their parents during the session in the counselor's presence. Also, the clients asked their friends or family to comment on their improved speaking when they noticed stuttering-free speech.

Public-Display

The client was instructed to seek out those circumstances or words or people that had been previously avoided because of their greater likelihood of producing stuttering and to speak in those circumstances using the prescribed procedures.

Post-Treatment Practice

The client was instructed to use the prescribed procedures continually and, further, to practice the new breathing pattern at regular times each day.

Follow-up

The counselor telephoned the client about three times during the first week to provide encouragement and to answer questions and called intermittently thereafter to obtain the reports of progress in addition to providing encouragement. The conversation by the client during these calls also gave the counselor direct information regarding the occurrence of stuttering.

Recording, Reliability and Validity

Before treatment, the client was asked to provide as accurate an estimate as possible of the average number of stuttering episodes per day he had been experiencing. After the counseling session, he recorded the number of stuttering episodes on prepared forms each day and gave the counselor the daily total during their follow-up telephone conversations. To validate this self-recording, the counselor contacted at least one friend or family member to corroborate the client's report of progress for 11 of the 14 clients. Similarly, the counselor recorded the number of times the client stuttered during the final telephone conversations with the client. For the two clients who had stuttered only on specific words, the counselor asked the clients to speak that type of word during the phone conversations.

RESULTS

Figure 6.2 shows the degree of stuttering after treatment expressed as a percentage of the pre-treatment level as recorded by the clients. The Figure shows that stuttering decreased by 94 per cent on the first day after treatment. On the second day, stuttering increased slightly but was still reduced by 90 per cent. Thereafter, stuttering became progressively less frequent reaching a 95 per cent reduction after 2 weeks, 97 per cent after 1 month, 99 per cent after 3 months and 93 per cent after 4 months. Since the clients were treated at different dates over a 7-month period, the 4-month data point is for 8 of the 14 clients. Two clients had been treated 8 months and 6 months previously.

The pre-treatment level was obtained just prior to treatment. The frequency after treatment was obtained from the record kept by the clients each day. The data points are expressed as a percentage of the client's pre-treatment level. Accordingly the pre-treatment level is 100 per cent. The

FIGURE 6.2. Frequency of stuttering for 14 clients

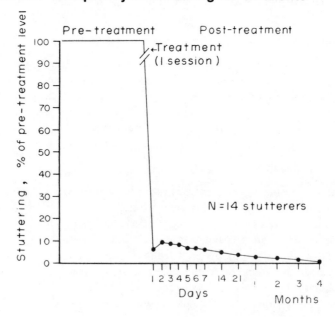

treatment occurred during a single 2-hr session designated by the slash mark at the arrow. Fourteen clients are included in all of the data through the first month; the fourth month includes eight clients. The data is given for each day of the first week, for each week of the first month, and monthly thereafter.

Analysis of the data of the individual clients showed that stuttering was reduced by at least 85 per cent for all clients on the very first day after treatment and by at least 93 per cent on the last follow-up day available for a client. Also, on the last available follow-up report, all reported that they stuttered so few times and so mildly that they no longer considered stuttering a problem for them. All reported that the stuttering episodes never occurred when they used the prescribed procedures. Because the stuttering episodes occurred only during the first few days, the forced interruptions in the speech pattern were similarly noticeable only during that period.

The two validating measures of the client's recording supported the general accuracy of the client's records. First, the comments of the client's family members to the counselor confirmed the low level, or total absence, of stuttering in every case. This confirmatory report was obtainable for 11 of the 14 clients.

The second validating measure was the client's speech over the phone with the counselor during the post-treatment inquiries and was obtained from all clients. In every case, the client's phone conversation was almost, or totally, free of stuttering. During the last follow-up phone conversation with each client, of about 10 min duration, the counselor had recorded the number of stuttering instances. For 13 of the 14 clients, no instance of stuttering occurred (as shown in the last column of Table 6.1). To make this measure more meaningful for the 2 clients who stuttered only on very specific words, the counselor required the 2 clients to use many instances of that type of word during the test conversation. Rather ironically, the only client who stuttered during the "test" phone conversation did so only at the very start of the conversation. He explained that he was so eager to tell the counselor about his delight over his progress, that he momentarily became too distracted to pause in his speech and to regulate his breathing in the manner he had been doing otherwise.

A general comment made by the clients and their family members was that the client now entered into conversations more frequently and no longer avoided persons or situations that had previously provoked stuttering. The clients also generally reported that great effort and resolve was needed during the first few weeks to adhere to the new speaking pattern but after the first few weeks, the new manner of speaking became automatic.

DISCUSSION

The new procedure was effective in reducing stuttering. The treatment was very rapid as seen by the 94 per cent reduction in stuttering on the very first day. The treatment was exceptionally brief as seen by the use of only one counseling session of 2 hr duration plus several follow-up telephone calls. The benefit endured for as long as follow-up information was available which was as long as 8 months for one client and 1 month for all clients at the time of this writing. The benefit was substantial for every client as seen by the reported absence of stuttering for eight of the clients and a reduction of 80 per cent or more for each of the other six clients at the end of one month. The treatment was effective for clients who stuttered very severely (one thousand episodes per day) as well as for the client who stuttered rarely (two episodes per day) but distressingly when speaking her name. Stuttering had been an enduring and severe problem for all clients as seen by the average of 24 yr of stuttering prior to treatment, and previous professional treatment. The treatment therefore appears to be applicable to the general range of severity of stuttering. All clients requesting and following the treatment were benefitted.

The method does appear to require great motivation and effort as seen by the reports of the clients that they had to concentrate consciously and continually during the first few weeks on their new manner of speaking and breathing. Also, the clients reported that the more consistently they used their new method when they felt at ease, the easier it was to remember to breathe and speak correctly when they were nervous or tense.

The present procedure appears to be more effective clinically than existing clinical methods. None of those methods have been reported to achieve as great a reduction as the present method (99 per cent) nor for as many clients (100 per cent) following the instructions, nor as rapidly (1 day), nor within such brief treatment (a 2-hr session), nor for such a long period (8 months).

REFERENCES

Azrin N. H., Jones R. J. and Flye B. (1968) A synchronization effect and its application to stuttering by a portable apparatus. *J. Appl. Behav. Anal. 4*, 283-295.

Azrin N. H. and Nunn R. G. (1973) Habit reversal: A method of eliminating nervous habits and tics. *Behav. Res. & Therapy 11*, 619-628.

Barber V. (1940) Studies in the psychology of stuttering XVI. Rhythm as a distraction in stuttering. *J. Speech & Hearing Dis. 5*, 29-42.

Beech H. R. and Fransella F. (1968) *Research and Experiment in Stuttering.* Pergamon Press, Oxford.

Fransella F. (1967) Rhythm as a distractor in the modification of stuttering. *Behav. Res. & Therapy 5*, 253-255.

Goldiamond I. (Personal communication).

Ingham R. J. and Andrews G. (1973) Behavior therapy and stuttering: A review. *J. Speech & Hearing Dis. 38*, 405-441.

Jacobson E. (1938) *Progressive Relaxation.* University of Chicago Press, Chicago.

Jones R. J. and Azrin N. H. (1969) Behavioral engineering: Stuttering as a function of stimulus duration during speech synchonization. *J. Appl. Behav. Anal. 2*, 223-229.

7

MOTOR

INTRODUCTION

Seizure Disorders

"Epilepsy" describes a heterogeneous group of disorders caused by disturbances in the electrical activity of the brain. Epilepsy may result from such factors as lesions, trauma, perinatal injuries, infections, and metabolic disorders, and is reported to have a base rate of 1 in 200 (Kolb, 1968). Seizure activities in children may vary from "momentary absences" frequently accompanied by petit mal symptoms, through grand mal epilepsies, to the massive convulsions of status epilepticus, which can result in death. Most seizures are preceded by a distinct "aura," which children frequently describe as a "funny feeling in the stomach." Specialists in epilepsy recognize the importance not only of adherence to the medication regimen but also of the effects of home, school, and social life on the seizure potential of the child or adolescent. In particular, compliance with medical treatment can be substantially affected by many factors. Carter and Gold (1968) suggest that fully 50 percent of epileptic children do not benefit from medication; Schmidt and Wilder (1968), in a more optimistic report, suggest that 70 to 80 percent of children do benefit from medication.

Clearly, the epileptic syndrome creates a major management issue for the various professionals who treat these children and their families. Effective treatment typically involves a team effort, requiring not only a medical specialist in epilepsy, typically a neurologist, but also a mental health professional, usually a social worker, who, with the physician can work with the family and the personal dynamics that affect adherence to the medical and psychological treatment regimens.

A subset of childhood epilepsies, the reflex epilepsies, which have a base rate of approximately 5 percent of all seizure cases, are elicited by a particular stimulus or stimulus complex. Much of the research on epileptic children, using behavioral techniques, has been on reflex epilepsy cases. These young patients often have their seizures precipitated by light, sound, touch, reading, or various self-stimulatory behaviors. Thus, environmental conditions may be a major factor in potentiating or attenuating the seizure disorder.

Feldman and Ricks (1978) have suggested that behavior therapists, seeking to intervene with epileptic children, have three major targets: the specific environmental trigger that sets off the attack, the reinforced behavior that occurs as a consequence of the attack, and the emotional state of the child, which may have precipitated the seizure. To those targets, one might add the children's cognitions and attributions developing when the attack occurs, as well as the attributions of peers, teachers, and parents.

In a review of the behavioral literature, Mostofsky and Balaschak (1977) classify treatments into three categories: reward and punishment, self-control, and psychophysiological techniques. Reward management typically requires that the occurrence of a seizure is not followed by excessive care, concern, or attention other than what is required for the safety of the child, while punishment programs may take the form either of placing a child in a time-out room or on a special care ward after seizure activity. Aversive experiences such as shouting, overcorrection, and even electric shock have been used with these children. Both overt and covert reward programs have been used, along with thought stopping and role playing. Self-control programs have included traditional progressive relaxation, as well as various hypnotic and imagery techniques combined with relaxation procedures. In self-control programs, children have been taught to record and to monitor their behavior, particularly preseizure behavior.

To understand antecedents of seizure behavior, Feldman and Paul (1976) have video-taped their patients before and during the seizure activity. Through a replay technique utilizing a split-screen, they have been able to study not only the seizure activity, but the in-patient's reactions to it. This method is perhaps helpful, but one must question the patient's personal reactions to observing his total loss of control. Forster and Campos (1964) have used progressive relaxation and systematic exposure to increasing degrees of various stimuli that elicit epileptic attacks. Forster (1977) has demonstrated the effectiveness of systematic desensitization in reducing response to seizure trigger stimuli, but he has not shown it to be equally effective with all areas. Certain epilepsies may be preceded by a complex of stimuli rather than by a single precipitant stimulus. Clearly, a more detailed analysis of antecedent behaviors is indicated.

Gardner (1967) has shown the role that modeling behavior may play in the development of a psychogenic seizure disorder as well as the effects of altering intrafamilial reinforcement contingencies. In this case, the child received reinforcement for behaviors incompatible with an epileptic seizure and nonreinforcement for seizure-like activity. The ten-year-old girl was treated by her parents who participated in three parent-teaching sessions on a weekly basis, and were instructed how to ignore her seizures and to reinforce more appropriate behaviors. Many seizure disorders, even those that are most clearly organic in nature and perhaps most refractory to a behavioral intervention, may have a learned component. To the extent that a learned component exists and that the behavior therapist does a thoughtful behavioral analysis, behavioral interventions may be possible. In the most difficult cases, behavioral interventions will, no doubt, be an adjunct to traditional medical intervention.

Zlutnik, Mayville, and Moffat (1975) present an excellent study in which aversive techniques were used to interrupt the behavioral chains leading to seizure activity. The "startle and shake" procedure was found effective in reducing overall seizure disorders to an acceptable level. A 9-month follow-up indicated that seizure levels remained acceptably low. Included in this chapter, by Ince (1976), is a case study of a 12-year-old child exhibiting both petit mal and grand mal seizures. A desensitization program was used to modify anxiety and a word cue association to eliminate seizures.

Cerebral Palsy

Cerebral palsy is a nonprogressive movement disorder resulting from intra-cranial defects due to injury or disease before, during, or after birth (Bakwin & Bakwin, 1972). Motor problems are frequently accompanied by sensory and perceptual defects that may create learning difficulties, severe emotional problems, and intellectual retardation. The incidence rate is approximately 3 per 1,000 of population in the United States, the rate being unaffected by economic, social, or geographical factors. Approximately one-third of these children have no potential for improvement while the upper third may never require services. Etiological factors can be divided into the prenatal, perinatal, and postnatal period with the latter two accounting for 80 percent of the defects. Genetic defects, prematurity, rubella, and related difficulties contribute to the prenatal causes. Premature birth is about six times as frequent among parents of cerebral palsied children than among the general population. Children with cerebral palsy are sometimes retarded in school development, and special educational arrangements are often necessary for their maximal rehabilitation. Sometimes they are unable to talk and must be taught to use language before locomotor training can be initiated.

Physical therapists face special problems requiring that they help these children develop reaching, grasping, and holding skills with the hands, as well as flexing, supporting, and moving skills of the legs to maximize whatever large and fine motor capabilities they may have. To achieve such skills, the child must have a high level of motivation and persistence. Additionally, workers with the cerebral palsied are concerned that these children maximize their ambulatory skills and control their weight sufficiently to allow them to move independently. Many of these children become heavier than their weak muscles can support. Work with these children requires a comprehensive, dedicated and multidisciplinary approach. In addition to the physician and physical therapist, the services of a dietitian, a behavior therapist, and other health professionals may be important.

Surprisingly little has been published in the research literature involving the application of behavioral techniques to the treatment of cerebral palsy and related motor disorders. Martin and Epstein (1976), in an excellent paper, surveyed the literature regarding therapeutic intervention with cerebral palsied patients and reported that there were few objective studies. They concluded that the limited amount of empirical research may be the result of a poor understanding of the symptoms of cerebral palsy and the design of ineffective treatment packages. Their paper also examined behavioral analysis procedures and experimental designs that are appropriate to the study of cerebral palsied children.

Rugel, Mattingly, Eichinger, and May (1971) report the study of an eight-year-old cerebral palsied child who was taught to place weight on his feet, causing a toy car to advance one space around the track. Back-up social reinforcers were also provided. When he slumped on his arms, consequently taking weight off his feet, reinforcement was withdrawn and the car moved backwards. This technique was effective in increasing the amount of time that the child would stand on his feet.

Loynd and Barclay (1970) report a shaping procedure to increase an eight-year-old girl's ability to stand and to take a few steps while grasping the table edge. She was gradually taught to pull up to the table, walk around it, and cross a short space to another table. The authors note such nonspecific treatment effects as increased responsiveness to her natural environment, along with spontaneous affectivity and an enhanced desire to learn other motor skills, such as self-feeding. Other studies report the use of behavior therapy to teach children to walk (Bank, 1968; Knapp, O'Neil & Allen, 1974; Chandler & Adams, 1972). Haavik and Altman (1977) reviewed the literature describing behavioral interventions that facilitated walking in retarded children, some of whom were also cerebral palsied. Horner (1971) presented an interesting study of a five-year-old mentally retarded spina bifida child who was taught to walk with the aid of crutches. The procedures used in this study are directly applicable to the treatment of similar difficulties with children who are primarily cerebral palsied.

Kolderie (1971) in her article in this chapter discusses specific behavioral techniques as they apply to the treatment of cerebral palsied children and presents a case illustrating how behavioral techniques can be used by physical therapists, occupational therapists, and speech therapists in collaborative treatment. Her study illustrates the type of comprehensive program necessary to maximize a cerebral palsied child's language, large motor, and fine motor skills. This article represents a good starting point for clinicians who are interested in such difficulties.

References

Bakwin, H., & Bakwin, R. M. *Behavior Disorders in Children*. Philadelphia: W. B. Saunders, 1972.

Bank, S. P. Behavioral therapy with a boy who had never learned to walk. *Psychotherapy: Theory, Research and Practice*, 1968, *5*, 150-153.

Carter, S., & Gold, A. Convulsions in children. *New England Journal of Medicine*, 1968, *278*, 315-317.

Chandler, L. S., & Adams, M. A. Multiply handicapped child motivated for ambulation through behavior modification. *Physical Therapy*, 1972, *52*, 399-401.

Feldman, R. G., & Paul, N. L. Identity of emotional triggers in epilepsy. *Journal of Nervous and Mental Disease*, 1976, *162*, 345-353.

Feldman, R. G., & Ricks, N. L. Nonpharmacologic and behavioral methods. In G. S. Ferriss (Ed.), *Treatment of epilepsy today*. Oradell, N.J.: Medical Economics Co., 1978, 89-111.

Forster, M. Reflex epilepsy. *Behavioral Therapy and Conditional Reflexes*. Springfield, Illinois: Charles C. Thomas, 1977.

Forster, M., & Campos, G. B. Conditioning factors in stroboscopic-induced seizures. *Epilepsia,* 1964, *5*, 156-165.

Gardner, J. E. Behavior therapy treatment approach to a psychogenic seizure case. *Journal of Consulting Psychology*, 1967, *31*, 209-212.

Haavik, S., & Altman, K. Establishing walking by severely retarded children. *Perceptual and Motor Skills*, 1977, *44*, 1107-1114.

Horner, R. D. Establishing use of crutches by a mentally retarded spina bifida child. *Journal of Applied Behavior Analysis*, 1971, *4*, 183-189.

Ince, L. P. The use of relaxation training and a conditioned stimulus in the elimination of epileptic seizures in a child: A case study. *Journal of Behavior Therapy and Experimental Psychiatry*, 1976, *7*, 39-42.

Knapp, M. E., O'Neil, S. M., & Allen, K. E. Teaching Suzi to walk by behavior modification of motor skills. *Nursing Forum*, 1974, *13*, 159-183.

Kolb, L. C. *Modern Clinical Psychiatry* (2nd ed.). Philadelphia: Saunders, 1968.

Kolderie, M. L. Behavior modification in the treatment of children with cerebral palsy. *Physical Therapy*, 1971, *51*, 1083-1091.

Loynd, J., & Barclay, A. A case study in developing ambulation in a profoundly retarded child. *Behaviour Research and Therapy*, 1970, *8*, 207.

Martin, J. E., & Epstein, L. H. Evaluating treatment effectiveness in cerebral palsy. *Physical Therapy*, 1976, *56*, 285-294.

Mostofsky, D. I., & Balaschak, B. A. Psychobiological control of seizures. *Psychological Bulletin*, 1977, *84*, 723-750.

Rugel, R. P., Mattingly, J., Eichinger, M., & May, J., Jr. The use of operant conditioning with a physically disabled child. *American Journal of Occupational Therapy*, 1971, *25*, 247-249.

Schmidt, R. P., & Wilder, B. J. *Epilepsy*. Philadelphia: F. A. Davis, 1968.

Zlutnik, S., Mayville, W. J., & Moffat, S. Modification of seizure disorders: The interruption of behavioral chains. *Journal of Applied Behavior Analysis*, 1975, *8*, 1-12.

THE USE OF RELAXATION TRAINING AND A CONDITIONED STIMULUS IN THE ELIMINATION OF EPILEPTIC SEIZURES IN A CHILD: A CASE STUDY

Laurence P. Ince

Summary—Following systematic desensitization treatment for anxiety associated with recurrent seizures, a combination of relaxation training and association of a cue word with the calm body state was employed to eliminate seizures in a 12-year-old boy with epilepsy. Following relaxation, the child was instructed to repeat the cue word several times so as to create a conditioned stimulus. After repeated pairings he was directed to verbalize the cue word to himself whenever he felt the aura of an approaching seizure. This resulted in avoidance of the onset of seizures and complete elimination of both grand mal and petit mal seizures. Long term follow-up showed no recurrence of seizures.

While some studies have been reported in which a behavioral technique has been employed for the reduction of seizures (e.g., Parrino, 1971), there is a general paucity of such work conducted either with seizures *per se*, or problem behaviors secondary to the primary diagnosis of epilepsy (e.g., Adams, Klinge and Keiser, 1973). The present report describes a case in which a child was treated for recurrent seizures through behavior modification methods.

CASE HISTORY

A 12-yr-old boy was brought for private treatment by his parents because of psychological problems associated with epilepsy of 4 yr duration.

Reprinted from *Behavior Therapy and Experimental Psychiatry*, 1976, 7, 39-42. Copyright 1976 by Pergamon Press, Inc. Reprinted by permission.
Laurence P. Ince is at Queens College of the City University of New York.

His parents reported that for four weeks prior to the initial therapy appointment he had been having numerous daily seizures in school, resulting in his being taken to the nurse's office where he would sleep for several hours. The seizures usually were of the petit mal type, but several grand mal episodes also had occurred. The school records indicated that petit mal seizures were characterized by the boy "blanking" out, i.e. staring into space without awareness of his environment and without responding to environmental stimuli for a duration of approximately 45-120 sec. Grand mal seizures were manifested as loss of speech, visual disturbances, falling, syncope and convulsive movements of his trunk and extremities. The duration of grand mal seizures typically was from 30-50 sec, following which he would fall asleep.

As a consequence of these episodes he had become fearful and reluctant to attend school. He felt that he "stood out" in school and had no friends, i.e. the other children teased him about his disorder and would not play with him. He began experiencing somatic problems, such as headaches, stomachaches and insomnia, which he used as excuses to remain at home, which his parents frequently permitted. In addition, he soon was to receive a new experimental medication with known possible detrimental side effects, and he was fearful about this.

According to his parents, the child's seizures had begun at the age of eight years, when epilepsy was first diagnosed, starting at nonsensical speech, catalepsy and facial tics. Prior to this time, his parents reported that he exhibited none of these symptoms and was in all respects a "normal, happy child." His disorder had progressed over the years to both the petit mal and grand mal seizures he was experiencing at the time his parents sought therapy for him.

At the time of his first interview he was receiving 200 mg of Dilantin® b.i.d. and 625 mg of Mysoline®t.i.d., and after the first week of therapy he began taking Tegretol® and Celontin® (exact dosages unknown). None of the medications were effective in controlling his seizures. His parents had consulted many neurologists and neurosurgeons over the years and had been told that there was diffuse hemispheric involvement (they could not recall which hemisphere) and that surgery was not possible.

With the exception of his epileptic disorder, the child was normal in all respects, was doing well academically and was a good athlete.

Treatment

Therapy initially focused on removal of the anxiety which the child experienced concerning school. Several hierarchies of anxiety-arousing situations were constructed with him. They included having seizures while in school and other public places, being ridiculed by other children, and receiving the new experimental medication. The hierarchies were as follows:

A. *Seizures in school*
   1. Sitting in a classroom and feeling an aura.
   2. The classroom environment begins to "fade away."
   3. A seizure begins.
   4. The teacher is speaking to him but he is unable to respond.
   5. Children and teacher gather around him.
   6. Seizure is out of control and he feels himself "blacking out."
B. *Seizure on baseball field*
   1. **Standing on pitcher's mound and feeling an aura.**
   2. People yelling at him to pitch but he is unable to do so.
   3. Other players, coaches, etc. gathering around him.
   4. Seizure begins and the environment "fades away."
   5. He falls and feels himself "blacking out."
C. *Being ridiculed by other children*
   1. Children laughing at him when he enters school.
   2. Children staring at him, pointing at him and laughing in his classroom.
   3. Children calling him names.
   4. Children telling him that he is "crazy," "retarded," etc., that he belongs in an institution.
   5. Children refusing to play with him or come to his house when he asks them to because he has epilepsy.
D. *Receiving the new experimental medication*
   1. Going with his mother to the physician.
   2. Physician gives his mother the medication and informs her of dosages.
   3. Physician warns him and his mother of possible negative side effects.
   4. At home, his mother calls him to receive his first dose.

Each hierarchy was treated during each therapy session. Progression was from the least anxiety-arousing item (1) to the most anxiety-arousing item on each list until the child was able clearly to visualize the final scene without experiencing any anxiety.

The child was trained in relaxation by a pseudo-hypnotic, suggestive tape recording (see Ince, 1970). A copy of the tape was made for him and he was instructed to practice relaxing at home at least twice per day. He also was instructed to relax himself at night, just before going to sleep, as a means of treating the insomnia. Relaxation was indicated to the therapist by the child raising a finger when he felt completely relaxed. When the child first began to relax his eyelids fluttered continually, but as relaxation progressed this gradually decreased and cessation of eyelid fluttering was used by the therapist as another indicator that he was relaxed. Complete relaxation was achieved within two therapy sessions and then systematic desensitization was started.

It required five therapy sessions, over a period of four and one-half weeks to eliminate the child's anxiety to the items. By the third session he reported considerably reduced anxiety and by the fifth session he stated that he no longer was "nervous" about any of the items. The somatic complaints no longer occurred and he was functioning normally in his various daily activities.

At this point it was decided to attempt a reduction of the child's seizures. He was relaxed completely twice during each therapy session. Once relaxation had occurred, he was instructed to say the word "Relax," 10 times, slowly. He also was told to practice the relaxation at home, as he had been doing, and when he felt himself to be deeply relaxed to say "Relax" slowly to himself 10 times. The rationale for this was explained to him, namely to associate a cue word with the relaxed body state so as to create a conditioned stimulus which could be used to produce the desired calm.

The child also was told to say the cue word to himself repeatedly whenever he felt the onset of a seizure approaching. This was possible since he invariably had a pre-seizure aura.

Therapy sessions were conducted once per week over a three-month period. The sessions were of approximately 60 minutes' duration.

Results

Table 7.1 presents the progress in seizure reduction. The information upon which the table is based was obtained from the patient, his parents, and school authorities. The first four weeks represent the pre-treatment period during which the child had between nine and 10 grand mal seizures and from 25-26 petit mal seizures per week. The pre-treatment period is the four weeks just before his first visit to the therapist. During the first five weeks of therapy, treatment was directed at alleviation of anxiety and there was only slight reduction in the rate of seizures. Therapy for seizure reduction began in the 10th week. There was an immediate reduction of both types of seizures to between one and two grand mal and between three and four petit mal seizures per week by the 13th week. By the 17th week, grand mal seizures were reduced to zero, petit mal episodes remaining at the low rate of 3 to 4 per week. The petit mal seizures were unchanged in frequency during the next four weeks, but grand mal episodes increased to between three and four per week.

The following month (weeks 22-25) the child went away to camp. According to him, and to his parents, who obtained their information from the camp physician, grand mal seizures remained as before during this time, but petit mal episodes increased slightly and his parents brought him home for one treatment session. This session was spent repeatedly relaxing the child

TABLE 7.1. Number of epileptic seizures per week

		Frequency	
	Weeks	Grand mal	Petit mal
Pre-treatment	1-4	9-10	25-26
Treatment for anxiety	5-9	8-9	24-25
Treatment for seizures	10-13	1-2	3-4
	14-17	0	3-4
	18-21	3-4	3-4
	22-25*	3-4	5-6
Follow-up	26-29	0	0
	30-33	0	0
	34-37	0	0
	38-63	0	0

*Patient seen for only one therapy session during this 4-week period.

and associating the cue word with the body state. He was instructed again on the importance of practicing this himself, which he admitted he had been lax in doing while at camp. Whenever he had had a seizure in camp, his counselors dealt with it in much the same way his teacher had, i.e. taking him to the physician's office where he would sleep.

From that time on he never experienced another seizure of either type. He was followed up through contact with his parents and with his school over the next three months, and both sources reported complete absence of seizures at home and in school. Resuming school in the fall did not increase the frequency of seizures. A report from the health authorities at the child's school six months later revealed that he had not had a single seizure, either grand mal or petit mal. There was thus a total of nine months without seizures since the termination of therapy.

DISCUSSION

Although this child had been receiving medications during the behavior therapy period, two of them, Dilantin® and Mysoline,® were drugs he had been taking for years, and which had not had an appreciable effect of his seizures. The Tegretol® and Celontin,® which he began taking after the first week of therapy (week 5 in Table 7.1) produced no significant reduction of seizures during the five weeks prior to the behavioral treatment. The new experimental medication previously mentioned was given to the child during the 18th week of therapy. It did not reduce the rate of seizures. Therefore, it is plausible that the behavioral technique of relaxation plus association of the cue word with the body state had produced the desired effects.

The behavioral correlates of relaxation were the child's indication to the therapist that he was relaxed by raising his finger, and cessation of eyelid fluttering. It is possible that complete muscle relaxation was not fully achieved. However, as Rachman (1968) has pointed out, reciprocal inhibition of anxiety may be accomplished if the patient achieves a state of calm. This certainly was true in the present case.

The child had been instructed to say the cue word to himself whenever he felt the approach of a seizure. He reported that he did this faithfully and that it resulted in the prevention of seizures. He stated that he would feel himself relax and felt the sensation of an approaching seizure "fade away."

It is difficult to determine precisely the role the child's parents played in the maintenance of his seizures. The possibility that they were reinforcing them must be considered. For example, when he had a seizure in school his father was notified immediately and he left work to get the child at school and take him home. Had the father been instructed not to rush to school when called, or the school nurse instructed not to call him when his son had a seizure, the frequency of the child's seizures might have been modified. However, since neither of these possibilities were realized their contingent effects must remain speculative. Although the parents were highly cooperative with regard to the behavioral techniques, all attempts to discuss with them their possible role in their son's problems were met with firm refusals.

The technique of relaxation plus cue-word association to create a conditioned stimulus may not be effective with all cases similar to the one presented herein, and such a generalization is not intended, particularly since total elimination of seizures is somewhat unusual. However, it does appear to be a worthwhile procedure to attempt with selected cases.

REFERENCES

Adams K. M., Klinge V. K. and Keiser T. W. (1973) The extinction of a self-injurious behavior in an epileptic child, *Behav. Res. & Therapy 11*, 351-356.

Ince L. P. (1970) Length of time required for relaxation in behavior therapy: A comparison of therapist and patient as relaxing agents. Paper presented at the Annual Convention of the American Psychological Association, Miami Beach.

Parrino J. J. (1971) Reduction of seizures by densensitization, *J. Behav. Ther. & Exp. Psychiat. 2*, 215-218.

Rachman, S. (1968) The role of muscular relaxation in desensitization therapy, *Behav. Res. & Therapy 6*, 159-166.

BEHAVIOR MODIFICATION
IN THE TREATMENT OF CHILDREN
WITH CEREBRAL PALSY

Mary L. Kolderie

A review of literature related to behavior modification as a treatment method is presented along with definitions of the terms used in behavior modification. Implications for the use of the methods in physical therapy are made, particularly as they relate to cerebral palsy. A case study is presented which describes how behavior modification was used by physical, occupational, and speech therapists in the treatment of a cerebral-palsied child. Conclusions are drawn which relate the specific programs given to basic principles of behavior modification.

During the past few years behavior modification has become a frequently used method of treatment for mentally retarded and psychiatric patients. Remarkable success with these patients has been reported. Although little has been written on the use of behavior modification in the treatment of cerebral palsy, this technique probably has much to offer in the training of children with cerebral palsy.

Behavior modification is a method of changing the overt behavior of an organism by using principles of learning theory. Simply stated, behavior modification may be defined as changing the rate at which an organism emits a response by administering a reinforcement after the response has been emitted.

Behavior modification is not a haphazard giving of rewards to a subject. Definite principles and techniques support the application of behavior modification. Michael and Meyerson state: "A behavioral approach to human control

Reprinted from *Physical Therapy* (Vol. 51:1083-1091, 1971). Copyright 1971 by the American Physical Therapy Association. Reprinted by permission.

Mary L. Kolderie is with Therapy Associates, Inc., Meguon, Wisconsin.

does not consist of a bag of tricks to be applied mechanically for the purpose of coercing unwilling people.

It is part of a highly technical system, based on laboratory investigations of the phenomena of conditioning, for describing behavior and specifying the conditions under which it is acquired, maintained, and eliminated."[1]

In behavior modification the emphasis is on observable actions of the subject. "A behavior system attempts to specify, without reference to unobservable, hypothetical inner-determining agents, the conditions and the process by which the environment controls human behavior."[1]

Gelfand and Hartmann list the following as essential aspects of a properly applied program of behavior modification.[2] First, a baseline of the behavior must be made by careful observation and recording. The treatment procedures must be described in specific detail. During therapy, continuous collection of data concerning the rate of emission of the behavior is essential. Reinforcement contingencies must be systematically varied in order to ascertain if the behavior is really under control of the therapist or is occurring by chance. The behavior that the therapist wishes to modify must be clearly and objectively defined and must be objectively measured. To evaluate the long range effects of the behavior modification program, a follow-up study should be done to see whether the behavior is persistent.

TERMS USED IN BEHAVIOR MODIFICATION

To facilitate a clearer understanding of the application of behavior modification, the following terms are defined.

Classical Conditioning

In classical or respondent conditioning, a stimulus elicits the response from the organism. If a neutral stimulus, that is, one that does not elicit the response, is paired with one that does, it acquires the power to elicit the response. The neutral stimulus then becomes a conditioned stimulus. The stimulus which initially does have power to elicit the response is called the unconditioned stimulus. The organism is reinforced by pairing the conditioned stimulus with the unconditioned stimulus. Classical conditioning is associated with reflex activity and with involuntary muscles.[3]

Operant Conditioning

In operant or instrumental conditioning, the organism must first make a response (perform an operation on the environment) before receiving a reinforcement. No stimulus elicits the response as in classical conditioning; however, a discriminative cue or stimulus that indicates to the organism when responses will be reinforced may be used. Most behavior modification programs fit into the operant conditioning paradigm.[3]

Reinforcement

Reinforcement is an event that changes the probability that a response will be emitted in the future. Reinforcers can be presented or withdrawn and the rate of responding can increase or decrease. A stimulus which does not change the rate of responding is not considered a reinforcer, but a neutral stimulus. Table 7.2 shows the various combinations of presentation or withdrawal and how each relates to changing the rate of behavior. Considerations of the behaviors of a child eating dinner serve as examples of the combinations in the table.

1. Presentation of a reinforcer increases the rate of desired behavior. The child eats all his food and receives a reinforcer of ice cream for desert.
2. Withdrawal of a reinforcer increases the rate of desired behavior. Mother nags at the child to eat his food. When the child eats, the mother stops nagging.
3. Presentation of a reinforcer decreases the rate of undesired behavior. Child spills his milk and is spanked.
4. Withdrawal of a reinforcer decreases the rate of undesired behavior. Child spills his milk and does not receive ice cream for dessert.

TABLE 7.2. Types of reinforcement

Response rate	Presentation of reinforcement	Withdrawal of reinforcement
	Positive Reinforcement	Negative Reinforcement
Response rate increases	Subject views reinforcement as pleasant. Reinforcement is given after subject responds.	An aversion stimulus is withdrawn when subject emits response.
	Punishment	Punishment
Response rate decreases	An aversion stimulus is presented after subject emits response.	A reinforcer, which subject views as pleasant, is withdrawn after subject responds.

Whether a reinforcer is pleasant or aversive must be defined by the effect it has on changing the rate of responding. Some stimuli used as reinforcers may be pleasant for some subjects, aversive for some and have no effect on others. A specific food is an example of such a stimulus.

In administering a behavior modification program, the specific reinforcer must be carefully selected. The reinforcer must appeal to the child.[4] A good idea is to try various reinforcers to see which is the most effective for the individual child. Examples of reinforcers for children are candy, ice cream, praise, being allowed to play with a favorite toy, and being allowed to engage in a desirable activity.

A primary reinforcer is a stimulus which has reinforcing power for the organism from the beginning. Examples are food, water, and electric shock. A secondary reinforcer is one that acquires power by being paired with a primary reinforcer. Examples are money, points, praise, and verbal disapproval. Often a behavior modification program will begin with pairing a primary reinforcer with a neutral stimulus. As the neutral stimulus acquires the power of a secondary reinforcer, the primary reinforcer is gradually eliminated.

Schedules of Reinforcement

Usually in the initial period of a behavior modification program, reinforcement is given on a continuous schedule—every response is reinforced. After the program is in progress, one of four types of intermittent schedules is used. In a fixed ratio schedule, a reinforcement is given after X number of responses. In a variable ratio schedule, the actual number of responses emitted before a reinforcement is given varies each time, but over a period of trials the average number of responses is X. In a fixed interval schedule, a reinforcement is given after Y amount of time has elapsed. (The subject must first emit a response to receive a reinforcement.) In a variable interval schedule, the time lapse between individual reinforcements varies, but on the average it is Y amount of time.[5]

Intermittent reinforcement has the following advantages; the behavior is not constantly interrupted by the subject partaking of his reinforcement (in the case of food or water), it yields higher rates of responding, and it becomes more resistant to extinction.[5] The transition from continuous to intermittent reinforcement must be gradual to prevent extinction from occurring during the nonreinforced trials.[5]

Regardless of the schedule of reinforcement, the reinforcement must follow the response as closely as possible in order that the organism learns that the reinforcement is contingent on a specific behavior.[4]

Extinction

When a behavior that has been reinforced is no longer reinforced, the frequency with which it is emitted decreases until the behavior is no longer emitted. This principle is used in behavior modification when the goal is to eliminate some undesirable behavior. To eliminate behavior in this manner, the therapist must first analyze the behavior to find what in the environment is reinforcing it. All reinforcement must be eliminated because partial reinforcement of the undesirable behavior will strengthen it.[3]

Behavior Shaping and Successive Approximation

Often the organism is not capable of emitting the final desired behavior; thus, if the experimenter waited for him to do so, the subject would never receive a reinforcement. The experimenter, therefore, reinforces a behavior which in some way resembles the final behavior. Each time he requires the behavior to be closer to the final behavior before giving the reinforcement. In this manner, the therapist guides or shapes the final behavior of the subject.[5]

Chains of Behavior

Many behaviors are complex, but can be divided into smaller components. One component of a chain is taught and reinforced first, then the other components are added to it before a reinforcement is given.[5]

Generalization of Behavior

If behavior modification is to have long lasting effects, the change in behavior must not become conditioned to the specific treatment situation. The subject must generalize the new or modified behavior to various situations where it is appropriate.[4]

Stabilization of Behavior

If the subject retains the new or modified behavior and does not regress to previous undesirable behaviors after the completion of the behavior modification program, the behavior has stabilized. To facilitate stabilization, intermittent schedules of reinforcement are used. To evaluate the stability of the behavior, studies should be done after a lapse of time.

Deprivation

Deprivation means that the subject has not received any of the specific reinforcers used in his training for a period of time. Frequently animals are deprived of food for twenty-four hours prior to training to ensure that they will be more motivated to work for food.[5]

Satiation

Satiation is the opposite of deprivation. When a subject is satiated, the frequency at which the behavior is emitted decreases. To avoid satiation of the child, the experimenter should use a variety of reinforcers or an intermittent schedule of reinforcement.

Baseline

Before the behavior modification program is initiated, a record is made of how frequently the behavior in question is emitted. The final rate of performance is compared with this baseline.

Reversal of Contingencies

In order to ensure that the change in the rate of behavior is the result of the behavior modification program, the reinforcement is varied from the desired behavior to the undesired behavior. If the rate of the desired behavior decreases and the rate of undesired behavior increases, the behavior modification is responsible for the change. The contingencies are then reversed to the desired behavior.[3]

BEHAVIOR MODIFICATION IN CEREBRAL PALSY

Denhoff and Robinault state: "Cerebral palsy is a manifestation or group of manifestations of impaired neurological function due to aberrant structure, growth, or development of the central nervous system."[6] They prefer the term *cerebral dysfunction* to cerebral palsy because it is a more inclusive term. Cerebral dysfunction may involve problems in any or all of the following areas: neuromotor, sensory, intellectual, behavioral, hearing, and sight.

Behavior modification can help children with cerebral dysfunction develop independence within the limits of their capabilities. It is not recommended as the only method to be used in the treatment of children with cerebral palsy; it should be used in conjunction with other methods. The application of behavior modification to the learning of motor skills and speech is described below.

Motor Skills

The development of motor skills is the area of greatest concern to the physical therapist in the habilitation of the child with cerebral dysfunction. In treating these children, one should emphasize abilities rather than disabilities. Denhoff and Robinault state: "It is well known that the full potentialities even of the normal individual are rarely, if ever, developed. In the presence of physical handicaps it is the wellspring of latent abilities that must be tapped if the patient is to realize to the full the life he is capable of enjoying."[6]

A well-administered behavior modification program has great potential for developing these latent abilities. Much of the training of motor skills in cerebral-palsied children depends upon motivating the child to develop his capabilities. The potential for performing the motor skill must be present before behavior modification can be effective in the development of this skill.

A nine-year-old mentally retarded girl was taught to walk by using food as a reinforcer.[7] Although the girl had no physical handicaps, she could not walk; impoverished environmental contingencies were believed to be responsible. Behavior was shaped first by having the child stand with assistance and then gradually progressing her to independent walking. After fifteen sessions of forty-five minutes each, she was able to walk by herself. Reevaluation six months later showed that the walking behavior had persisted.

A three-year-eight-month-old boy, who seldom engaged in physical activity but who was not physically handicapped, was conditioned to play on a large climbing-frame and to engage in other forms of physical activity.[8] The experimenters shaped the behavior by using reinforcers when the boy came near the frame. Verbal approval, smiling, and physical contact were used as reinforcers. After nine days of continuous reinforcement for climbing-frame behavior, the contingencies were reversed and climbing frame behavior dropped nearly to zero. The authors concluded that the behavior modification program was responsible for the increase in physical activity.

Harris and co-workers reported that they were able to extinguish crawling and reinstitute walking in a three-year-five-month-old girl.[9] The child was withdrawn and avoided all contacts with children, adults, play material, and equipment. She was normal physically and had walked at an earlier age.

The baseline observation showed that the child spent only 6.7 percent of her time on her feet. The reinforcement was to withold attention for off-feet behavior and to give attention for on-feet behavior. No punishment was given. After two weeks of continuous reinforcement for standing and walking, her activity level was like that of the other children in the nursery. A reversal of contingencies showed that the reinforcement was causing the change in the child's behavior. In addition, the child increased in verbal and social interaction with adults and peers. The authors concluded that "social reinforcement principles, carefully delineated and applied, can provide effective and efficient guidance tools for teachers and parents of young children."[9]

Typing skill was increased in an eighteen-year-old boy with traumatic quadriplegia.[7] Before the behavior modification program began, the patient did not persist in the job of typing. He frequently sought the therapist's attention and was reinforced for this by obtaining it. The behavior modification program consisted of placing him in a quiet room for typing, ignoring his demands for attention, and reinforcing him for thirty minutes of typing. The reinforcement was five minutes of conversation on a topic that interested him. As the program progressed, he was required to type a certain number of lines to be reinforced. If he did not persist in the task, he could not meet the criterion in thirty minutes. After twelve sessions, his rate increased from five to twelve lines in thirty minutes, and errors decreased from three per line to one every other line.

Meyerson and co-workers reported success in teaching a seven-year-old boy with cerebral palsy to walk.[7] The physician and the physical therapist thought that the boy actually was able to walk without assistance. They believed that he had a fear of falling which was being maintained by receiving attention. Behavior was shaped by placing him between two chairs so that he could hold onto the backs of the chairs. Gradually the chairs were moved farther apart so that the boy had to walk to get from one chair to the other. He was reinforced with tokens which could be exchanged for toys. After five days he was walking independently and was reinforced by the natural contingencies of the freedom which independent walking has.

In addition he was taught to fall correctly by using tokens to reinforce his behavior. The authors concluded: "It is perhaps sufficiently noteworthy that an important behavior that had been unobtainable previously by traditional physical therapy methods was obtained in just four sessions of 20 minutes by utilizing the principles of behavior theory. Moreover, the behavior was engaged in willingly, almost eagerly, and with little or none of the emotionalism that the subject was reported to have shown in previous attempts to teach him to fall."[7] They also stated: "The rapidity with which the falling behavior was obtained lends some support to the belief that tokens functioned as strong generalized conditioned reinforcers."

Unwanted motor behavior is characteristic of many children with cerebral palsy. If they are to function successfully in a motor task, they must be able to control involuntary movements.

MacPherson described how he conditioned a sixty-year old woman with Huntington's chorea to control involuntary movements.[10] First, she was trained in relaxation techniques. Next, silver wire electrodes were implanted under the skin over muscles which had involuntary contractions. The wires were connected to earphones. She was instructed to try to relax her muscles as soon as the auditory signal indicated that an involuntary contraction was beginning. The method was successful. The patient resumed a fairly normal gait and was able to perform activities without as much interference from involuntary movements as she had had previously.

Patterson used candy, pennies, and peer group approval to condition a nine-year-old hyperactive child with cerebral dysfunction to concentrate on his work in school.[11] The child's hyperactive behavior decreased markedly after a few days of conditioning. His activity level became similar to that of normal children. Patterson stated that the crucial idea in eliminating hyperactive behavior was to give immediate reinforcement for socially acceptable behavior which was incompatible with the hyperactive behavior. He also mentioned the importance of stimulus generalization in the elimination of hyperactive behavior. Conditioning sessions should occur in a wide variety of situations.

Many of the authors who were cited mentioned that they used the principle of shaping in the conditioning of a motor skill. In the training of children with cerebral palsy, the importance of shaping of behavior cannot be emphasized enough. The therapist must reduce the motor task to component parts and determine what skills are necessary in order to perform the desired motor task. These components and the preliminary skills should be ranked in order of difficulty. The therapist then begins training at the highest level that the child can perform easily. As the child's performance improves more of the components are required of him before a reinforcement is given until, finally, he can perform the entire motor skill.

Speech

The goals of speech therapy are to eliminate old patterns, to form new associations, and to establish correct sounds in speech. Exercises of speech muscles and functional activities such as sucking and licking are commonly used to help children overcome their speech difficulties.[6] Behavior modification has a role in the treatment of children whose problem is primarily organic because the child still needs to be motivated to use what he can to the best of his ability.

Cook and Adams state: "Speech deficiency may be viewed as failure of coordination of stimulus and response function. Speech deficiency may be a function of inadequate learning . . . or it can be a product of reinforcing contingencies."[12] In some cases, the individual may have learned inappropriate responses and relearning, or a more stringent control of reinforcing stimuli, may be a solution to speech deficiency. They emphasize the necessity of discovering the conditions that will lead to the emission and development of appropriate responses. Such conditions are not sufficiently available for the speech deficient child in the normal environment; thus, the structured environment of a behavior modification program is desirable for these children.

Lovaas and others taught autistic children to speak using the principle of shaping.[13] Correct verbal behavior was reinforced with food. Incorrect verbal behavior was never punished. After the children learned many words, they were taught to use them. The authors thought that the immediate food reinforcement was the crucial variable in the child's learning. Behavior modification was used with some success on a seven-and-one-half-year-old autistic boy.[14] Initially he could mimic television commercials but did not have functional use of language. By using candy as a reinforcer, he was taught words, parts of speech, and sentences. Kerr and co-workers reported that they were able to teach a mute three-year-old girl, who was mentally retarded and had cerebral palsy, to make vocalizations by using social reinforcements.[15]

Most of these studies mentioned above concern autistic children rather than children with cerebral palsy. Although the causes of the problems differ, the goals of learning to make sounds, producing sounds correctly, putting sounds together into words, and understanding and using words correctly in communication are common to both types of children. The success that the previously cited authors have had with the application of behavior modification on children with speech difficulties suggests that it may be a worthwhile method for children with cerebral palsy.

CASE STUDY

The following case study is an example of how behavior modification was used in the treatment of a ten-year-old girl with cerebral palsy.

Medical History

CS, a full-term baby weighing three kilograms, was born on July 1, 1959. During delivery, she had suffered cord strangulation for twelve minutes and had not begun to breathe until thirty minutes after the initiation of resuscitory measures. She had not cried or sucked until two weeks after birth. She was admitted to the Children's Rehabilitation Center at the University of Minnesota in March 1966 with the following diagnoses: severe athetosis secondary to prolonged hypoxia at the time of birth, mild spastic diplegia, and severe speech problems. She was probably of average intelligence.

At the time of admission CS had a vocabulary of thirty words, only ten of which were understandable to strangers. She had difficulty eating, and drooled frequently. She was beginning to learn to crawl and could walk with much assistance. With the aid of side rails, she could attain the sitting position and, once sitting, she could maintain position unassisted. Assistance was needed with all hand activities such as dressing, washing, and eating. Range of motion and strength of all extremities were normal, but coordination was poor. Her hearing was normal, but she lacked conjugate eye movements. Psychological tests administered in April 1966 indicated that CS was above average in general conceptual ability and average in verbal and mathematical ability. She had poor spatial ability and visual form discrimination which is indicative of a perceptual problem.

CS was put on a poker chip reward system in September 1966 in an attempt to alleviate her eating problems and to increase her enthusiasm. Chips and washers were used in speech, occupational therapy, physical therapy, and on the ward. The chips and washers could be exchanged for candy or toys.

Physical Therapy

The goal of physical therapy for CS was independent ambulation with crutches and short leg braces. When treatments were begun, she could roll over with difficulty, sit and balance on hands and knees with great difficulty. She could not crawl or balance in the kneel-standing position.

The program began with the development of skill in rolling over and sitting up, then progressed to balancing and crawling on hands and knees, and finally to balancing on her feet and walking. Immediate verbal reinforcement was given for performance of these skills. Washers were given after the activity when the therapist's hands were no longer needed to assist the child. Each day a higher level of performance was required to obtain a reinforcement.

CS achieved the objectives of independence in crawling, balancing on the hands and knees and in the kneel-standing position for a long period of time, and walking short distances on her knees. Standing balance with crutches is the current goal. She is able to stand independently for two to three minutes with short leg braces and weighted forearm crutches. She is not able to walk independently with the crutches, but can walk with the assistance of another person.

Occupational Therapy

In occupational therapy CS practiced hand activities to increase strength and coordination of her upper extremities. One example was the grasping, holding, and releasing of a wooden cylinder 15 centimeters long and 2.5 centimeters in diameter. Records were kept of how long CS could hold the cylinder. She was reinforced for each increase in time. The initial reinforcer was a washer. During a two-month period, the time which she could hold the cylinder increased from twenty to one hundred seconds. Gradually the reinforcement was shifted to natural contingencies until CS was reinforced by increased skill in holding her crutches.

CS enjoyed typing on an electric typewriter. If she was diligent with her exercises, she was allowed to type two days a week for one-half hour; hence, typing served as a reinforcement as well as a useful activity to learn. Records were kept of her progress in speed and accuracy in typing. Perceiving her own recorded progress was also reinforcing.

Speech Therapy

CS had difficulty eating and talking because of the weakness of her tongue and lips. Speech therapy began with a feeding program to strengthen her weak muscles. She was reinforced for correct eating behavior and later for correct pronunciation of sounds. Initially, she received washers or chips, then points. As CS's pronunciation improved, she was required to make a certain number of correct responses within a time limit to receive a point. Next, she was required to correctly use the sound in syllables and words to be reinforced. Thus, the principle of shaping was used. Records of CS's progress in speech were kept. The records themselves served as a reinforcer for her.

The speech therapy program was continued at home, and her parents were instructed in what sounds to identify and reinforce with points. When she had earned five hundred points, she was rewarded by a shopping trip and dinner in a restaurant. Social reinforcement replaced points or chips. Reinforcement came through talking to people and having them understand her and converse with her.

The goal in speech therapy had been the acquisition of skill in producing correctly all sounds in the English language and in being able to use them in conversation. She began with a vocabulary of thirty words, most of which were not understandable. Her vocabulary increased to that of an eight-year-old child, with 75 to 80 percent of the words being understandable.

Before CS began receiving speech therapy her parents were quick to interpret her gestures and sounds, which discouraged any further attempt at speech. Behavior modification was important in providing the necessary incentive for CS to learn to speak.

Conclusion

The case study does not intend to prove that behavior modification is better than other methods of treatment. Because behavior modification was used throughout CS's habilitation program and because a reversal of contingencies was not done, one cannot conclude that behavior modification was a crucial variable in her improvement.

The case report does demonstrate many of the principles used in behavior modification. The principle of shaping and programming of the skills to be learned was used throughout CS's habilitation program. The report also shows how a variety of reinforcers can be used. CS was reinforced with washers and chips, points, praise, and by being allowed to engage in a desired activity. The importance of immediate reinforcement was stressed throughout her program.

An important aspect of the program was shifting from the artificial reinforcers of washers and points to natural reinforcing contingencies. Behavior which is being maintained only by the artificial contingencies of a behavior modification program is likely to extinguish when the program ends. Natural reinforcers, therefore, are needed to maintain the behavior after the program has been completed. CS received natural reinforcement for correct speech by being understood. She was reinforced for doing her exercises by being able to engage in the activities she desired, such as standing with her crutches and doing more with her hands.

SUMMARY

Behavior modification has been successful in the treatment of mentally retarded, autistic, and psychiatric patients. It has been a motivating factor in changing the behavior of these patients. Behavior modification has great potential as an adjunct in the habilitation of children with cerebral palsy.

REFERENCES

1. Michael J, Meyerson L: A behavioral approach to counseling and guidance. *Harvard Ed Rev 32*:382-402, 1962.
2. Gelfand DM, Hartmann DP: Behavior therapy with children: A review and evaluation of research methodology. *Psychol Bull 69*:204-215, 1968.
3. Ullmann LP, Krasner L: *Case Studies in Behavior Modification.* New York, Holt, Rinehart and Winston, 1965, pp 1-65.
4. Werry JS, Wollersheim JP: Behavior therapy with children. A broad overview. *J Amer Acad Child Psychiat 6*:346-370, 1967.
5. Holland JG, Skinner BF: *The Analysis of Behavior.* New York, McGraw-Hill, 1961, pp. 41-203.
6. Denhoff E, Robinault IP: *Cerebral Palsy and Related Disorders. A Developmental Approach to Dysfunction.* New York, McGraw-Hill, 1960, pp. 1-57, 67-85, 197-202.
7. Meyerson L, Kerr N, Michael JL: *Behavior Modification in Rehabilitation.* In *Child Development: Readings in Experimental Analysis,* edited by Sidney W. Bijou and Donald M. Baer. New York, Appleton-Century-Crofts, 1967, pp 214-239.
8. Johnston MK, Kelley CS, Harris FR, et al: An application of reinforcement principles to development of motor skills of a young child. *Child Develop 37*:379-387.
9. Harris FR, Johnston MK, Kelley CS, et al: Effects of positive social reinforcement on regressed crawling of a nursery school child. *J Ed Psychol 55*:35-41, 1964.
10. MacPherson ELR: Control of involuntary movement. *Behav Res Ther 5*: 143-145, 1967.
11. Patterson GR: *An Application of Conditioning Techniques to the Control of a Hyperactive Child.* In *Case Studies in Behavior Modification,* edited by Leonard P. Ullmann and Leonard Krasner. New York, Holt, Rinehart and Winston, 1965, pp. 370-375.

12. Cook C, Adams HE: Modification of verbal behavior in speech deficient children. *Behav Res Ther 4*:265-271, 1966.
13. Lovaas OI, Berberich JP, Perloff BF, et al: Acquisition of imitative speech by schizophrenic children. *Science 151*:705-707, 1966.
14. Weiss HH, Born B: Speech training or language acquisition? A distinction when speech training is taught by operant conditioning procedures. *Amer J Ortho-psychiat 37*:49-55, 1967.
15. Kerr, N, Meyerson L, Michael J: *A Procedure for Shaping Vocalizations in a Mute Child.* In *Case Studies in Behavior Modification*, edited by Leonard P. Ullmann and Leonard Krasner. New York, Holt, Rinehart and Winston, 1965, pp. 366-370.

8

SLEEP

INTRODUCTION

Sleep-onset Insomnia

Insomnia refers to any condition in which inadequate sleep is obtained. Sleep-onset insomnia involves an inordinately long time between "bedtime" and sleep onset. Almost all children, especially during preschool years, experience this problem to some degree (Inglis, 1976). If the problem becomes chronic through inadvertent parental reinforcement, or the child has excessive ruminations about inability to sleep, then clinical help may be needed. Traditional medical treatments have utilized hypnotic drugs. However, a recent review of behavioral treatments points out several reasons why pharmacological intervention is undesirable (Ribordy & Denney, 1977). Children usually develop a tolerance for the drug in a few weeks; side effects can include morning drowsiness, nausea, or headache. Use of drugs may alter sleep patterns, decreasing rapid eye movement (REM) sleep (dreams), which may be needed for psychological health. When the drugs are withdrawn, excessive REM sleep may occur, along with nervousness, increased insomnia, and even nightmares. Finally, children may come to believe that they can fall asleep only with the drug; this belief may interfere with ability to sleep after drug withdrawal.

The behavioral approach to insomnia relies on relaxation and imagery procedures to reduce excessively high levels of arousal and ruminations prior to sleep. Progressive relaxation can reduce the overall muscle tonus, and result in a feeling of deep relaxation conducive to sleep (Borkovec, Kaloupek, & Slama, 1975). If children complain of worrisome thoughts at bedtime, training in pleasant imagery to replace those thoughts can be helpful.

Other treatments for insomnia include stimulus control and paradoxical intention (Turner & Ascher, 1979). In stimulus control therapy, only sleep behaviors are allowed to occur on the bed so that the bed becomes a discriminative stimulus for sleep. In paradoxical intention, the patient is told to stay awake as long as possible. This eliminates an anxiety about trying to go to sleep. Neither procedure has been tried with children.

Weil and Goldfried (1973) demonstrated the use of relaxation procedures in the treatment of an 11-year-old girl's insomnia. In this study, it was determined that the girl's insomnia was not related to attention-seeking behavior reinforced by the parents. Importantly, the first session of relaxation training took place in the child's bedroom, and was performed by the therapist. This allowed the child to apply what she learned in the appropriate setting and let the therapist check on the child's response to relaxation instructions. The use of tape-recorded instructions after the first session allowed therapy to continue with minimal therapist contact. Interestingly, the child's ruminations at bedtime subsided and other positive changes were observed in her behavior during the day.

Nocturnal Problem Behaviors

Problem behaviors that prevent adequate sleep and can be bothersome to parents include the child's demands for attention, either before going to bed or after reported nightmares. The child may have a fear of the dark or of being alone, and desire parental companionship. By refusing to sleep or to stop crying until the parent agrees to stay with the child during sleep, an otherwise normal child can learn to modify the parents' behavior to the point that they always attend to the child. In a similar manner, the child's reporting of nightmares may be reinforced to the point that the parents feel the child has serious psychological disturbance. This disorder may be assisted with other behavioral problems in feeding, elimination, or social skills development caused by the child's manipulation of the parent's behavior (Klatskin, Jackson & Wilkin, 1956). Traditional treatments such as psychoanalysis or logical reassurance have been relatively ineffective (Wright, Woodcock & Scott, 1970).

The behavioral approach includes extinction of reinforcement by parental attention, and social reinforcement of improved sleeping patterns the morning after. The child is given a time earlier in the evening for parental attention, and attention just before bedtime is eliminated. Inglis (1976) reports several case studies in her review. In one case, a child's incessant crying had been reinforced by the parents allowing her to sleep with them. Treatment involved ignoring the child's screaming, and resulted in normal sleep patterns in two weeks. Bergman (1976) reported a similar case in which a seven-year-old boy kept his parents awake until they let him come into their bedroom. The pediatrician had diagnosed the boy as hyperactive, and this supposedly explained the child's activities at night. Behavioral treatment involved ignoring the child's disturbances and never allowing him to sleep with his parents. The problem behavior, which had persisted over a long period, was eliminated in two weeks, and daytime "hyperactivity" was reduced.

In the study of sleep disturbance by Wright, Woodcock, and Scott (1970) included in this chapter, a preschool girl who had not had a full night's sleep in two years displayed a normal sleep pattern after 35 days of treatment. The parents provided extra attention before bedtime, and ignored crying and pro-tests from the child. Typically, the child's expressed fears of the dark were eliminated. Since the parents did not respond to the expressions of fear, the child had to face the night alone, and soon became desensitized to the nocturnal environment. This study is noteworthy because sleep problems were eliminated using behavioral techniques in a child who was thought to have organically based hyperactivity from minimal brain damage.

REFERENCES

Bergman, R. L. Treatment of childhood insomnia diagnosed as "hyperactivity." *Journal of Behavior Therapy and Experimental Psychiatry*, 1976, *7*, 199.

Borkovec, T. D., Kaloupeck, D. G., & Slama, K. M. The facilitative effect of muscle tension-release in the relaxation treatment of sleep disturbance. *Behavior Therapy*, 1975, *6*, 301-309.

Inglis, S. The nocturnal frustration of sleep disturbance. *MCN: American Journal of Maternal Care Nursing*, 1976, *1*, 280-287.

Klatskin, E. H., Jackson, E. B., & Wilkin, L. C. The influence of degree of flexibility in maternal child care practices on early child behavior. *American Journal of Orthopsychiatry*, 1956, *26*, 79-93.

Ribordy, S. C., & Denney, D. R. The behavioral treatment of insomnia: An alternative to drug therapy. *Behaviour Research and Therapy*, 1977, *15*, 39-50.

Turner, R. M., & Ascher, L. M. Controlled comparison of progressive relaxation, stimulus control, and paradoxical intention therapies for insomnia. *Journal of Consulting and Clinical Psychology*, 1979, *47*, 500-508.

Weil, G., & Goldfried, M. R. Treatment of insomnia in an eleven-year-old child through self-relaxation. *Behavior Therapy*, 1973, *4*, 282-294.

Wright, L., Woodcock, J., & Scott, R. Treatment of sleep disturbance in a young child by conditioning. *Southern Medical Journal*, 1970, *63*, 174-176.

TREATMENT OF SLEEP DISTURBANCE
IN A YOUNG CHILD BY CONDITIONING

Logan Wright
James Woodcock
Robert Scott

Sleeping problems frequently are encountered in early childhood, especially between the ages of one and five.[1] Their range includes night terrors (pavor nocturnus), nightmares, bedwetting, and resistance to going to bed. Research into the etiology of such problems has been limited and speculative. Anthony[2] has concluded that sleeping disturbances are likely to have two factors in common, a suggestible child and certain stressful environmental conditions (such as precocious exposure to aggression or sex). The manifestations are thought to be determined by the physiologic predisposition of the child. For example, if a child is visually hypersensitive, the sleeping problem probably will be one of hallucinations and nightmares. In the psychoanalytic literature, sleeping problems in the child are considered a manifestation of the child's fears. The fear may be of separation from parents, of losing control, or of what may happen while asleep. The origin of such anxieties is thought to lie in psychosexual, developmental conflicts. Sleep problems are often related to seizure activity and to cerebral dysfunction in general.[2, 3]

Although relatively little is known about the causes of sleep disturbance there has been even less research in the treatment of such problems. Logical reassurance of the child is believed by Kessler[4] to do no good. The typical

Reprinted from *Southern Medical Journal*, 1970, *63*, 174-176. Copyright 1970 by Southern Medical Society. Reprinted by permission.

Logan Wright is in the Department of Pediatrics and the Children's Memorial Hospital, University of Oklahoma Medical Center. James Woodcock is in Melville, New York, and Robert Scott is at the Veterans Administration Hospital, Miami, Florida.

psychoanalytic approach involves analysis of the child aimed at helping him to "work through" the conflict which necessitates the symptom.[5]

In recent years the technics of behavioral modification (conditioning and extinction) have been successfully applied to behavioral problems similar to sleep disturbance. Problems successfully treated by conditioning technics include: tantrums,[6] head bumping,[7] crying,[8] psychogenic seizures,[9] and hyperactivity.[10, 11] When the patient discussed in this report was first called to our attention, it seemed logical that a conditioning approach might be effective in this childhood sleeping problem. This notion was supported by the work of Murray[3] who thinks that social learning can be responsible for creating sleep patterns, and refers to the treatment of adult insomnia by progressive relaxation, a behavioral modification technic. Furthermore, a conditioning approach was suggested by the work of Williams[6] who has applied extinction procedures to control nap and bedtime temper tantrums of a 20 month old boy whose behavior was felt to be solely an attention getting mechanism. The present study relies on both extinction and procedures of need reduction to control what was presumed to be a combination of organically based hyperactivity, phobic display, as well as tantrum and attention getting behavior.

REPORT OF A CASE

The patient, a 3 year 8 month old girl, had been adopted at 6 days of age. She had the first seizure at 10 months, and since then has had mild seizures at intervals of several months. Neurologic examination at the age of 3 years led to a medical impression of minimal brain damage, probably of the nature of a seizure disorder manifested by minimal hemiatrophy, increased tendon reflexes and an abnormal EEG record (slowing, primarily in the left temporal region).

The patient's sleep disturbance commenced at approximately 2 weeks of age. She began to cry for long periods from early in the evening until early the next morning. As she became older, the crying was mainly when being put to bed. She would cry, scream and kick her bedroom door. An apparently phobic element appeared in the form of repeated protests that spiders were in her room, and in the contention that she could see and feel them. Tantrums and phobic displays at bedtime typically lasted approximately 90 minutes. She would also awaken several times nightly and repeat her protests for brief periods. The patient reportedly had not slept over 5 hours continuously at any time over the past 2 years.

Her response to medication had been unsatisfactory. She had marked hyperactivity following barbiturates as well as after dextroamphetamine and methyphenidate hydrochloride. She became overly sedated when given acetazolamide or diphenylhydantoin. Prednisone and chloral hydrate partially alleviated the hyperactivity and seizure activity, though neither helped the sleeping problem. At the time of our study the patient was not on medication, except that prednisone was available to be administered by her mother in the event of a seizure.

Before conditioning was begun, the parents had attempted several methods of coping with the patient's nocturnal protests. These included reasoning, criticism, and physical punishment. The usual pattern was the parents' refusal to allow the child out of her room, threatening and reasoning with her through the door. On occasions they would let her sleep with them if she would stop crying. It is impossible to determine the exact role of organic factors in precipitating and maintaining the child's sleeping problem. However, at the time conditioning was begun organicity appeared to account for a small percentage of the difficulty. Emotional behavior in the form of attention seeking and phobic reaction appeared to be the major factor interfering with sleep.

Primary responsibility for carrying out the conditioning program was vested with the parents. First, they agreed to provide the child with one hour of undivided attention immediately before her designated bedtime. This was an attempt to reduce the patient's inordinate desire for attention, which seemed to constitute one aspect of the drive which was producing her protests. Secondly, the child's parents agreed to place her in bed each night at 8:30 PM, and were to say pleasantly, "Good night, we'll see you in the morning." They agreed to leave the room, lock the door and not reenter the room or communicate with the child until after 7 o'clock the next morning. These latter procedures were in an attempt to extinguish the nocturnal protests which had been reinforced by the attention gained when the parents responded with reasoning, criticism, threats, spanking, allowing the patient to sleep with them, etc. A record was kept of the number and duration of protests each night, beginning with the day on which the conditioning program was begun.

One of us was present in the home during the child's attention period and for approximately 1 to 2 hours after she was placed in bed on the first 3 evenings of the program. After the first 3 days we did not visit the home, but consulted with the mother and recorded progress during weekly one hour sessions. Active treatment under our supervision lasted 10 weeks.

Results

The patient's behavior showed immediate improvement. The number of protests at bedtime decreased markedly and outbursts during the night ceased almost completely. The total time spent in protesting went from 90 minutes on the day before conditioning (which the parents reported was an approximate average time for all days prior to conditioning) to 15 minutes on each of the first 2 days of the conditioning program. There were only 5 days between day 3 and day 35 where the patient protested for longer than a total of 5 minutes. Since day 35, there have been no reports of any difficulty. These data are shown in Figure 8.1.

On the 5th night of the study, the parents left the patient in charge of a babysitter. On that night she reportedly cried for approximately 15 minutes. During the 2nd week of the study the patient resorted to turning on the light in her bedroom. The following week the lightbulb was removed and she reportedly cried for approximately 30 minutes on one occasion and for 45 minutes on another. During the 5th week of treatment the patient had seizures on 2 successive days. Her bedtime was not affected on these 2 days, but on the following day she cried for 45 minutes. A follow-up inquiry was made of the parents 10 weeks after our active supervision had ceased. They reported the patient was sleeping undisturbed for 10 to 11 hours each night without crying or protest behavior at bedtime.

DISCUSSION

It is felt that the above results support the effectiveness of conditioning procedures in modifying a childhood sleeping problem. By combining an extinction technic (patient locked in a room without being able to receive attention from her parents) with an attempt to reduce the need for attention which was apparently motivating the patient's protests, a severe and long-lasting problem of bedtime protesting and phobic behavior, which were incompatible with sleep, was quickly brought under control.

It should be stressed that the patient's failure to sleep apparently did not result solely from either of the three items: attention getting behavior, phobic responses, or organically based hyperactivity. On the one hand it is more understandable how the conditioning program used in this case may have influenced her attention getting and phobic behavior rather than hyperactivity resulting from an organic involvement. By providing attention before bedtime, but never afterward, the patient's attention getting behavior was apparently extinguished. By continually forcing her to confront fear which was not realized and thus not reinforced, the patient apparently became desensitized to this problem. On the other hand the effect of the conditioning program on the organically based hyperactivity is less and this is understandable, since it is possible that such hyperactivity was no longer a factor in the patient's sleep problem at the time conditioning was begun.

Too often in the past, the suspicion of an organic diagnosis, such as brain dysfunction, has precluded therapeutic intervention. Yet studies by Patterson[10] and by Pihl,[11] utilizing conditioning procedures to reduce what was presumed to be organically based hyperactivity, are encouraging. The present study supplements these data by suggesting that behavior problems which may accompany cerebral dysfunction, particularly where organicity is

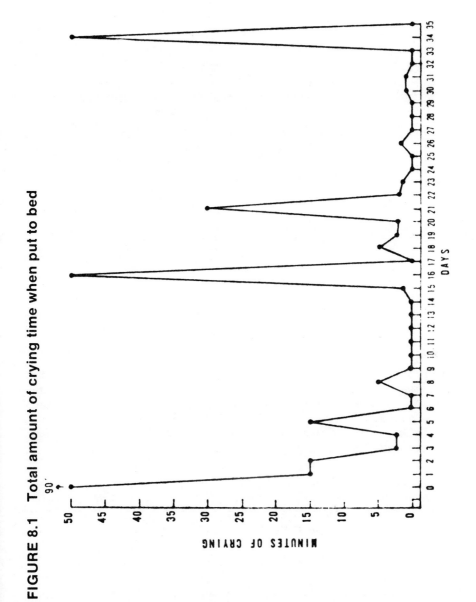

FIGURE 8.1   Total amount of crying time when put to bed

thought to be a precipitating but not sole cause of the disturbance, can be treated successfully by means of conditioning technics. These data also serve as a replication of Williams'[6] work which suggests tantrums and other emotional behaviors at bedtime can be extinguished.

REFERENCES

1. Gesell, A., and Ilg, F.: *Infant and Child in the Culture of Today.* New York, Harper and Row, 1943.
2. Anthony, J.: An experimental Approach to the Psychopathology of Childhood Sleep Disturbances, *Brit J Med Psychol 32*:19, 1959.
3. Murray, E. J.: *Sleep, Dreams and Arousal.* New York, Appleton-Century-Crofts, Inc., 1965.
4. Kessler, Jane: *Psychopathology of Childhood.* New Jersey, Prentice-Hall, Inc., 1965.
5. Fraiberg, Selma: On the Sleep Disturbances of Early Childhood. *Psychoanalytic Study of the Child.* New York, International Universe Press, Inc., 1950.
6. Williams, C. D.: The Elimination of Tantrum Behavior by Extinction Procedures, *J Abnorm Soc Psychol 59*:269, 1959
7. Mogel, S., and Jeriff, W.: Extinction of Head-Bumping Symptoms of Eight Years Duration in Two Minutes. A Case Report, *Behav Res Ther 5*:131, 1967.
8. Hart, Betty M., Allen, K. Eileen, Buell, Joan S., Harris, Florence R., and Wolf, Montrose: Effects of Social Reinforcement on Operant Crying, *J Exp Psychol 1*:145. 1964.
9. Gardner, J. E. : Behavior Therapy Treatment Approach to a Psychogenic Seizure, *J Consult Psychol 31*:209, 1967.
10. Patterson, G. R.: A Learning Theory Approach to the Treatment of the School Phobic Child. In Ullmann, L. P., and Krasner, L. (Eds): *Case Studies in Behavior Modification.* New York, Holt, Rinehart and Winston, 1965, p. 257.
11. Pihl, R. O.: Conditioning Procedures with Hyperactive Children, *Neurology 17*:421, 1967.

9

RESPIRATORY

INTRODUCTION

Bronchial asthma is a condition characterized by difficult breathing due to constriction of the bronchial airways. Patients may show symptoms of labored breathing, shortness of breath, coughing and wheezing, and anxiety due to fears of suffocating. Sixty percent of persons who have asthma are under 17 years of age (Purcell & Weiss, 1970). Most are boys. Asthmatic children represent a heterogeneous group with respect to the variety of factors that can cause this syndrome (Purcell, 1975). Allergies, infections, and emotional responses to ailments are generally identified as stimuli that precipitate attacks. Asthmatics may be roughly dichotomized into those for whom a clear environmental precipitant can be identified and those for whom no clear antecedent irritant, allergen, or emotional state is apparent. Any of four emotional reactions may commonly precede asthmatic attacks: anger, excitement with pleasurable feelings, anxiety, and depression (Walen, Hauserman & Lavin, 1977). Most researchers recognize the importance of exploring the effect of affective states and cognitions in precipitating asthmatic symtoms. In this disease there is a close interaction between the psychological and the physiological. Clearly, certain children, particularly those who are atopic or who have an early history of colicky behavior, show a greater sensitivity to allergens and other environmental irritants. Liebman, Minuchin, and Baker (1974) suggest that the family plays a substantial role in the maladaptive social learning that may occur around asthmatic attacks.

It has been estimated that four to five million people in the United States suffer from this malady (Purcell & Weiss, 1970). Long-term studies indicate that approximately 50 percent outgrow asthma; only 10 percent will have severe symptoms after 20 years (Ellis, 1975). Though asthma may be a life-threatening disorder, the fatality rate is reported to average about 1.5 per thousand asthmatics (Mustacchi, Lucia, & Jassy, 1962). Despite the fact that the mortality rate may be relatively low, the quality of life that the asthmatic child or adolescent experiences can be greatly diminished due to the psychological and behavioral repercussions of this disorder.

Behavioral treatment of asthmatic children usually involves the following: a) reducing the effectiveness of antecedent conditions that elicit the asthmatic attack; b) training the child in progressive relaxation techniques and various cognitive procedures to reduce anxious responses to the symptoms; c) training the parents in affective responding to the asthmatic attacks along with strengthening incompatible and independence-encouraging behaviors; and d) training the young patient in compliance to medication and other treatment procedures. Additionally, hypnosis and biofeedback procedures have been used to train bronchial dilation. Purcell and Weiss (1970), in their article reviewing factors that affect asthmatic behavior, suggest that assessment involve a detailed interview with parent and child, along with behavioral observations in the natural environment. The parent and family are encouraged to assist in the development of a list of triggering stimuli for asthmatic conditions to determine antecedents. These antecedents are then ranked in order of importance and their relative duration and frequency determined. The patient is next asked to provide a detailed history of a recent asthmatic attack. From this history one can determine whether the difficulty is primarily one due to antecedents, perhaps amenable to a respondent therapy, or one maintained by the consequences, amenable to operant procedures. In any case, a detailed behavioral analysis is important.

In an excellent article, Knapp and Wells (1978) reviewed 24 studies involving the behavioral treatment of asthmatic children and adults. From their review they conclude that the respondent techniques of relaxation training and systematic desensitization can produce statistically significant improvements in respiratory functioning of asthmatic children, while operant techniques present an equivocal picture. They advocate the study of compliance to medical procedures and the use of self-control techniques.

The behavioral treatment of asthma may be divided into three categories: contingency management, punishment techniques, and relaxation therapies and biofeedback. Lukeman (1975) presents the case of a four-year-old asthmatic who began to develop a wheeze while attending nursery school. An examination of the mother's and school personnel's responses to her wheezing showed that they could reinforce this behavior with attention. The mother then was instructed in ways of altering the consequences of these attacks by not removing her from the playroom and encouraging the staff to involve her in activities. Within three weeks the wheezing cleared up. Neisworth and Moore (1972), in their article included in this chapter, illustrate the use of parental management of contingencies with a seven-year-old asthmatic boy. After receiving instructions in operant conditioning, the mother analyzed her own behaviors and concluded that she had been quite effective in reinforcing his asthmatic responses, particularly those occurring just before bedtime. An extinction procedure was used to avoid reinforcing bedtime asthmatic attacks. At the same time a program of reinforcement of incompatible behaviors was developed. An 11-month follow-up showed no return of behaviors.

Renne and Creer (1976) present a two-part study of children trained to use the Intermittent Positive Pressure Breathing (IPPB) device, which delivers bronchial dilator medication to the lungs under positive pressure. Through prompting, shaping, and reward behaviors of eye fixation, facial posturing, and diaphragmatic breathing, using a multiple baseline design, four children were trained to use the IPPB apparatus. Follow-up revealed that use of the device reduced the amount of follow-up treatment and medication necessary for more optimal control of asthma. The results of their second study suggest that nursing personnel can be easily and effectively trained to implement such behavioral programs.

Creer (1970) demonstrates the use of punishment techniques in treating two ten-year-old boys who had a history of repeated admissions to the hospital for asthmatic attacks. Preliminary analysis revealed that the boys found the hospital setting highly reinforcing. It was hypothesized that the children purposely brought on asthmatic attacks by hyperventilation and by not seeking medical attention during the early stages of the attacks. On admission to the hospital the boys were placed in separate private rooms and permitted to leave only for eating and trips to the bathroom, and staff contact and privileges such as use of television and comic books were restricted. This time-out procedure was effective in reducing both the number of asthmatic-related hospital admissions and the length of time that the boys remained in the hospital.

References

Creer, T. L. The use of time-out from positive reinforcement procedures with asthmatic children. *Journal of Psychosomatic Research*, 1970, *14*, 117-120.

Ellis, E. F. Allergy disorders. In V. Vaughn & R. J. McKay (Eds.), *Nelson textbook of pediatrics*. Philadelphia: Saunders, 1975.

Knapp, T. J., & Wells, L. A. Behavior therapy for asthma: A review. *Behaviour Research and Therapy*, 1978, *16*, 103-105.

Liebman, R., Minuchin, S., & Baker, L. The use of structural family therapy in the treatment of intractable asthma. *American Journal of Psychiatry*, 1974, *16*, 165-168.

Lukeman, O. Conditioning methods of treating childhood asthma. *Journal of Child Psychology and Psychiatry*, 1975, *16*, 165-168.

Mustacchi, P., Lucia, S. P., and Jassy, L. Bronchial asthma: Patterns of morbidity and mortality in the United States. *California Medicine*, 1962, *96*, 196-200.

Neisworth, J. T., & Moore, F. Operant treatment of asthmatic respondings with the parent as therapist. *Behavior Therapy*, 1972, *3*, 95-99.

Purcell, K., & Weiss, J. H. Asthma. In C. G. Costello (Ed.), *Symptoms of psychopathology*. New York: John Wiley & Sons, Inc., 1970, 597-623.

Purcell, K. Childhood asthma: The role of family relationships, personality and emotions. In A. Davis (Ed.), *Child personality and psychopathology: Current topics* (Vol. 2). New York: Wiley Interscience, 1975, 101-135.

Renne, C. M. & Creer, T. L. Training children with asthma to use inhalation therapy equipment. *Journal of Applied Behavior Analysis*, 1976, *9*, 1-11.

Walen, S. R., Hauserman, N. M., & Lavin, P. J. *Clinical guide to behavior therapy*. Baltimore: Williams and Wilkins, Co., 1977.

OPERANT TREATMENT OF ASTHMATIC RESPONDING WITH THE PARENT AS THERAPIST

John T. Neisworth
Florence Moore

Pronounced reduction of chronic asthmatic responding in a 7-year-old boy was achieved through parental management of "therapeutic" contingencies. Treatment was begun with professional guidance by the mother after she had attended several instructional sessions in operant conditioning. Reinstatement of original consequences and return to treatment contingencies produced corresponding changes in the duration of asthmatic behavior. An 11-month follow-up confirmed the stability of the therapeutic changes, general improvement in the child's health, and the absence of any demonstrable deleterious side-effects. The results suggest closer and extended scrutiny of operant techniques in the treatment of asthma and other allergic responses.

Applying empirically based principles and strategies, behavior therapies are increasingly promoting the feasibility and desirability of using the home as the setting and parents as the agents for child therapy. This is in contradistinction to traditional approaches that employ hypothetical models, clinical settings, and highly trained personnel.

A growing number of successful studies dealing with various child problems is demonstrating the economy of time and professional effort of behaviorally based therapies. Representative of such studies are those of

Reprinted from *Behavior Therapy* 1972, *3*, 95-99. Copyright 1972 by Academic Press, Inc. Reprinted by permission.

John T. Neisworth is in the Department of Special Education at Pennsylvania State University. Florence Moore is with the Wilmington Special School District, Wilmington, Delaware.

Williams (1959), O'Leary, O'Leary, and Becker (1967), and Zeilberger, Sampen, and Sloane (1968) dealing generally with parental treatment of disruptive or aggressive child behaviors. Lal and Lindsley (1968), and Conger (1970) provide examples of somatic problems responsive to therapy conducted by mothers. Results and descriptions of training groups of mothers as reinforcement therapists are reported by Lindsley (1966), and Hirsch (1968).

The problem of interest in this study, asthma, has received much attention from psychoanalytic perspectives but rarely has asthma been conceived of as an operant (see review by Hirt, 1965). Turnbull (1962) has summarized previous research that views asthma as a learned response. Most of this research, however, has employed a respondent rather than operant paradigm. While asthma-like responses can be respondently conditioned, extinction rapidly occurs in the absence of UCS, and it is suggested that operant reinforcement could account for maintenance and amplification of respondently or organically produced asthmatic responses. While this study does not investigate the origin of asthmatic responses in a child, it does report successful treatment through operant procedures.

HISTORY AND DIAGNOSIS

The patient, a 7-year-old boy, was the oldest of two sons of American parents who resided in Japan until the patient was 18 months old. At the age of 6 months, the boy was diagnosed as asthmatic; he was frequently hospitalized for periods of 1-4 weeks. Doctors stated that his condition would probably improve upon the family's return to the United States. However, by the age of two the patient continued to display repeated asthmatic attacks (coughing, wheezing, abrupt inspiration) which required frequent visits to the hospital emergency room for immediate relief. From the ages of 2 to 7 years, the boy was seen almost monthly by a specialist due to continued severity of the problem. Various medications were administered and dietary restrictions imposed in an effort to ameliorate the condition.

Results of the various medical attempts were questionable; the child still had frequent attacks and visits to hospital emergency rooms remained necessary.

By the time it was suggested that the child might be helped by behavior therapy, a pattern of parental concern and continued attention to the problem had been well established. Typically, the mother would caution the child not to overexert himself, not to eat certain foods, and to be sure to take his medicine. She described the child as "nervous" and reported that emotional upsets or excitement precipitated the child's attacks. Of particular concern were the child's prolonged wheezing and coughing at bedtime. Further investigation revealed that both medicine and sympathetic attention were given especially during the bedtime asthmatic episodes.

After exposure to operant conditioning rationale and treatment procedures, the mother herself suggested that the child's problem might well be conceived of in operant terms and treated accordingly. She analyzed her own behavior towards the child and suggested that it might be supporting or aggravating the problem. Specifically, it was hypothesized first, that asthmatic responding was being maintained or amplified by the presentation of verbal and tactile attention (as well as medicine) during or immediately after a seizure, and second, that behavior incompatible with coughing, wheezing and generally "being sick" was not being reinforced. A schedule of differential reinforcement for being "sick" as opposed to being well seemed to be operating.

INTERVENTION AND RESULTS

In addition to the case history, and prior to any systematic changes in the contingencies related to asthmatic behaviors, data were collected for 10 days to provide a baseline (Figure 9.1). It was decided to record only nighttime in-bed responding since this was the occasion of most intense behavior; further, it was not possible to obtain accurate daytime data. Due to the nature of the responses and data collection restrictions, duration rather than frequency was chosen as the response measure. Coughing, wheezing, gasping, and similar responses lacking in discreteness and often overlapping in occurence made frequency counts difficult. Response time, however, was relatively easy to record. All data were collected each evening in the home of the child by the junior author.

Immediately following the baseline phase, two systematic treatment strategies were initiated. First, based on the hypothesis that parental attention to the problem was reinforcing the behavior, an extinction procedure was employed. The parents agreed to discontinue all attention and administrations of medicines during bedtime asthmatic attacks. The child was put to bed with the usual affectionate interactions between parents and child. Once the bedroom door was closed, however, no further interaction occurred until morning.

Because extinction procedures often require extended use, it was decided to implement an additional strategy, reinforcement of incompatible behavior. Specifically, the child was told he could have lunch money (instead of taking his lunch to school) if he coughed less frequently on a given night than the night before. This contingency permitted reinforcement for even slight improvements in the behavior, making reinforcement highly probable and progress easy.

It can be seen from Figure 9.1 that the initial effect of the intervention program was to increase the duration of coughing and wheezing. (We have frequently found this initial inflation of behavior on an extinction schedule.) However, after 7 days the effects of treatment became noticeable; by Day 23 the behavior reached a low that remained somewhat stable.

To provide further evidence of the efficacy of the treatment contingencies, the parents relucantly agreed to reversal procedures. Specifically, attention and medication again were given during the brief asthmatic episodes. (Lunch money, however, was not withdrawn, i.e., the child received money on a noncontingent basis.) As Figure 9.1 shows, response duration increased quickly and climbed towards baseline intensity. At this point, the parents urged a return to the treatment contingencies. This was done, resulting again in an initial increase in response duration followed by a drop to a stable new low of about 5 min. As a follow-up, the parents periodically were requested to time bedtime coughing. This reminded the parents of the need to continue the new contingency arrangements and provided follow-up data. During 11 months of such follow-up inquiries and data, the problem remained at essentially the treatment low (between 2-7 min).

FIGURE 9.1. Duration of bedtime asthmatic responding as a function of contingency changes

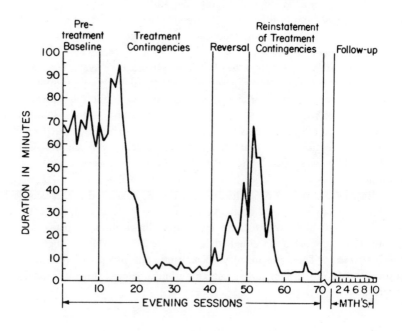

DISCUSSION

The systematic management of two simple contingencies resulted in a drastic reduction in the duration of nighttime asthmatic responding in a 7-year-old boy. Withholding of attention during coughing and wheezing and "payment" for reduction of such responding successfully and quickly effected changes that years of medical treatment alone could not. Reinstatement of the original cough-attention contingency relationship produced a return to prolonged asthmatic episodes. Minimal responding was again established upon restoration of treatment contingencies. An 11-month follow-up failed to reveal any appreciable increment in the child's nighttime asthmatic attacks. Indeed, the parents reported that daytime coughing also sharply declined and pediatrician's reports indicated a general improvement in health. This study, which adds to the growing literature that stresses the crucial role of "therapy" conducted by parents, does not purport to obviate "organic" factors in the etiology or maintenance of asthmatic responses. Rather, it pinpoints the dramatic role that environmental contingencies may have in the amplification and attenuation of the problem.

REFERENCES

Conger, J. C. The treatment of encopresis by the management of social consequences. *Behavior Therapy*, 1970, *1*, 386-390.

Hirt, M. L. *Psychological and allergic aspects of asthma.* Springfield, IL: Charles C. Thomas, 1965.

Hirsch, I. S. Training mothers in groups as reinforcement therapists for their own children. *Dissertation Abstracts*, 1968, *28* (11-B), 4-156.

Lal, H., & Lindsley, O. R. Therapy of chronic constipation in a young child by rearranging social contingencies. *Behavior Research and Therapy*, 1968, *6*, 484-485.

Lindsley, O. R. Parents handling behavior at home. *Johnstone Bulletin*, 1966, *9*, 27-36.

O'Leary, K. D., O'Leary, S., & Becker, W. C. Modification of a defiant sibling interaction pattern in the home. *Behavior Research and Therapy*, 1967, *5*, 113-120.

Turnbull, J. W. Asthma conceived as a learned response. *Journal of Psychosomatic Research*, 1962, *6*, 59-70.

Williams, C. D. The elimination of tantrum behavior by extinction procedures. *Journal of Abnormal and Social Psychology*, 1959, *59*, 269.

Zeilberger, J., Sampen, S., & Sloane, H. N. Modification of a child's problem behaviors in the home with the mother as therapist. *Journal of Applied Behavior Analysis*, 1968, *1*, 47-53.

10

ELIMINATION

INTRODUCTION

Enuresis

Enuresis is defined as the involuntary discharge of urine in the absence of neurological or urologic pathology. Diurnal enuresis refers to wetting that occurs when the child is awake; nocturnal enuresis, the more common, to wetting when the child is asleep. Enuresis is generally considered to be a problem when it occurs in a child older than three or four years of age. About 88 percent of enuretics stop wetting by the age of four and a half years, 90 percent by seven and a half years, and almost all the rest by 17 years (Pierce, 1972). About twice as many boys as girls are enuretic. The problem is more common with children from lower socioeconomic classes. Although two types have sometimes been distinguished—primary enuresis, that is, by children who have never demonstrated continence, and secondary enuresis, by children who have been continent for a period of several months before regressing to nighttime wetting—these classifications are not particularly useful to the clinician for treatment of the problem.

It has been estimated that more than 50 different drugs and methods have been used to treat enuresis (Campbell, 1970). Anticholinergics, antidiuretics, psychotropic drugs, imipramine hydrochloride, hormones, and CNS stimulants have all been tried with varying degrees of success. Psychoanalysis tends to regard enuresis as a symptom of some other underlying disturbance and treatment is aimed at dealing with the "real" problem rather than the wetting. Self-hypnosis (Olness, 1975) and dietary restrictions (McKendry, Stewart, Khana, & Nettig, 1975) have also been tried. However, none of these approaches has been as effective as direct behavioral approaches for treating the problem.

One of the most successful behavioral techniques for treating nocturnal enuresis has been the bell and pad apparatus, based on the work of Mowrer and Mowrer (1938), and a modification using two buzzers developed by Lovibond (1964). Reviews of these respondent conditioning techniques (Doleys, 1977; Jones, 1960; Lovibond, 1964; Werry, 1966; Yates, 1970; Young, 1965) suggest 75-90 percent initial success for those treated. Relapse rate is about 41 percent, with most of the relapses occurring within six months of treatment; when relapsed children are retreated, the success rate is about 68 percent. Several companies sell a bell and pad apparatus under names such as "Wee Alert." The apparatus includes two foil pads, with holes in the top pad, separated by an absorbent sheet, which are placed under the child's lower bed-sheet and connected to a box containing two six-volt batteries, a sensitive relay, and a buzzer. As soon as the child begins wetting, the circuit is completed and the loud buzzer sounds awaken the child (and the whole household). Once awake, the child shuts off the buzzer, goes to the toilet and empties his bladder before returning to bed. Dry nights are usually rewarded with small amounts of money, gold stars on a chart, a toy, a record, or some other reinforcer. Well-run studies (Baker, 1969; DeLeon & Mandell, 1966) suggest that this method is superior to traditional psychotherapeutic techniques, with no evidence of symptom substitution.

Enuresis is also treated using operant techniques. Based on the idea that bladder tension serves as a stimulus for urination and that children who urinate in bed do so under conditions of only slight tension, Kimmel and Kimmel (1970) developed a daytime shaping procedure for enuretic children, teaching them to delay urination for increasingly longer periods. Praise and tokens redeemable for trinkets are used as reinforcers for delaying urination, and the technique has been reported to be successful in relatively short periods of time (Kimmel & Kimmel, 1970; Paschalis, Kimmel, & Kimmel, 1972; Stedman, 1972).

The article presented in this chapter describes a remarkable multifaceted treatment program called "Dry Bed Training" developed by Azrin, Sneed, and Foxx (1974). Their program combines a number of techniques, including cleanliness training, private practice, nighttime awakening, retention control, and positive rewards, into a rapid, intensive training procedure. The program requires close monitoring through the night, and is probably best conducted by a professional trained in the procedures rather than by parents. It is an extremely effective treatment program, requiring only one night of intensive training involving hourly awakenings of the child, followed by less intensive supervision until seven consecutive dry nights have passed. Dry bed training is an excellent procedure for many enuretic children, particularly those who have been unsuccessful with other procedures. Either it or, if a trained professional is not available, the bell and pad apparatus is highly recommended.

Encopresis

Encopresis is defined as repeated fecal soiling after three years of age when not due to organic pathology. Discontinuous encopresis refers to children who have had a period of continence but who have relapsed; continuous encopresis, to those who have soiled regularly since infancy. The disorder is about four times more common in boys than girls. About 1.5 percent of normal seven-year-old children are encopretic.

Like that of enuretics, treatment of encopretics has ranged from drugs (such as imipramine) to psychoanalysis. Behavioral treatment programs have used both classical and operant conditioning techniques. Young (1973) taught encopretic children to associate gastroileal reflexes with the toilet situation. He instructed parents to give a warm drink or food to the child when awakening in the morning. After 20 to 30 minutes, the child was taken to the toilet and a bowel movement suggested. The child then was asked to sit on the toilet for ten minutes and was praised for a bowel movement. This procedure was repeated daily as frequently as possible. Tablets of Senokot were also given at bedtime to aid in achieving bowel movement the next morning. Young found the technique to be effective with 19 of 24 children. Conger (1970) successfully treated a nine-year-old encopretic boy in one day by instructing his mother to ignore the boy after soiling and requiring him to clean himself. Others (Keehn, 1965; Pedrini & Pedrini, 1971; Gelber & Meyer, 1965) have structured social praise, candy, money, and tokens to bring about appropriate toileting.

The article in this chapter by Logan Wright (1973) gives an excellent description of how to deal with this problem. His four-step program has been highly successful with 35 out of 36 cases. He reports that he has follow-up data for as long as four years on some of his patients, all of whom have shown no relapse. A further study of 14 additional children was also highly effective (Wright, 1975). Using a procedure similar to Wright's, Christophersen and Rainey (1976) showed equally impressive results.

Constipation

Constipation refers to the infrequent evacuation of feces. It is a fairly common problem with children at various ages, most frequently caused by stool holding or refusing to sit on the toilet. Davidson, Kugler, and Bauer (1963) recommend hypertonic phosphate enemas given in pairs an hour apart for severe cases of constipation. Mineral oil is also prescribed, along with training to go to the toilet at regular times.

Lal and Lindsley (1968), the authors of the case study in this section, present an interesting description of a maladaptive behavior being unwittingly maintained by the child's mother who would entertain the boy in an attempt to entice him to pass stools. Withdrawing the attention of the mother and making playing in the tub contingent upon stool elimination quickly ended the constipation problem.

Summary

The above studies on behavioral treatment of enuresis, encopresis, and constipation illustrate the effectiveness of behavioral treatments for these disorders. Enuresis in particular has received an enormous amount of attention since the development of the Mowrer and Mowrer apparatus, which is probably the most thoroughly investigated procedure with children in the behavioral field (Christophersen & Rapoff, 1979). Behavioral treatment programs for this problem are highly effective. Few studies other than case reports exist on the behavioral treatment of encopresis and constipation. These problems are infrequently seen by the clinician, which might explain why so little research has been done on them.

REFERENCES

Azrin, N. H., Sneed, T. J., & Foxx, R. M. Dry-bed training: Rapid elimination of childhood enuresis. *Behaviour Research and Therapy*, 1974, *12*, 147-156.

Baker, B. Symptom treatment and symptom substitution in enuresis. *Journal of Abnormal Psychology*, 1969, *74*, 42-49.

Campbell, M. F. Neuromuscular uropathy. In M. F. Campbell & J. H. Harrison (Eds.), *Urology* (Vol. 2). Philadelphia: Saunders, 1970.

Christophersen, E. R., & Rainey, S. K. Management of encopresis through a pediatric outpatient clinic. *Journal of Pediatric Psychology*, 1976, *1*, 38-41.

Christophersen, E. R., & Rapoff, M. A. Behavioral pediatrics. In O. F. Pomerleau & J. P. Brady (Eds.), *Behavioral medicine: Theory and practice*. Baltimore: Williams and Wilkins, 1979.

Conger, J. C. The treatment of encopresis by the management of social consequences. *Behavior Therapy*, 1970, *1*, 386-390.

Davidson, M., Kugler, M. M., & Bauer, C. H. Diagnoses and management in children with severe and protracted constipation and obstipation. *Journal of Pediatrics*, 1963, *62*, 261-275.

DeLeon, G., & Mandell, W. A comparison of conditioning and psychotherapy in the treatment of functional enuresis. *Journal of Clinical Psychology*, 1966, *22*, 326-330.

Doleys, D. M. Behavioral treatments for nocturnal enuresis in children: A review of the recent literature. *Psychological Bulletin*, 1977, *84*, 30-54.

Gelber, H., & Meyer, B.   Behavior therapy and encopresis: Complexities involved in treatment.   *Behaviour Research and Therapy*, 1965, *2*, 227-231.

Jones, H. G. The behavioral treatment of enuresis nocturna. In H. J. Eysenck (Ed.), *Behaviour therapy and the neuroses*. New York: Pergamon Press, 1960.

Keehn, J. D.   Brief case report: Reinforcement therapy of incontinence. *Behaviour Research and Therapy*, 1965, *2*, 239.

Kimmel, H. D., & Kimmel, E.   An instrumental conditioning method for the treatment of enuresis.   *Journal of Behavior Therapy and Experimental Psychiatry*, 1970, *1*, 121-123.

Lal, J., & Lindsley, O. R. Therapy of chronic constipation in a young child by rearranging social contingencies. *Behaviour Research and Therapy*, 1968, *6*, 484-485.

Lovibond, S. H. *Conditioning and enuresis*. New York: Macmillan, 1964.

McKendry, J. B., Stewart, D. A., Khana, F., & Nettig, C.   Primary enuresis: Relative success of three methods of treatment.   *Canadian Medical Association Journal*, 1975, *113*, 953-955.

Mowrer, O. H., & Mowrer, W. M. Enuresis: A method for its study and treatment.   *American Journal of Orthopsychiatry*, 1938, *8*, 436-459.

Olness, K. The use of self-hypnosis in the treatment of childhood nocturnal enuresis. *Clinical Pediatrics*, 1975, *14*, 273-279.

Paschalis, A., Kimmel, H. D., & Kimmel, E.   Further study of diurnal instrumental conditioning in the treatment of enuresis nocturna.   *Journal of Behavior Therapy and Experimental Psychiatry*, 1972, *3*, 253-256.

Pedrini, B. C., & Pedrini, D. T.   Reinforcement procedures in the control of encopresis: A case study.   *Psychological Reports*, 1971, *28*, 937-938.

Pierce, C. M. Enuresis. In A. M. Friedman & H. I. Kaplan (Eds.), *The child* (Vol. 1). New York: Atheneum Publishers, 1972.

Stedman, J. M. An extension of the Kimmel treatment method for enuresis to an adolescent: A case report.   *Journal of Behavior Therapy and Experimental Psychiatry*, 1972, *3*, 307-309.

Werry, J. S. The conditioning treatment of enuresis. *American Journal of Psychiatry*, 1966, *123*, 226-229.

Wright, L. Handling the encopretic child. *Professional Psychology*, 1973, *4*, 137-144.

Wright, L.   Outcome of a standardized program for treating psychogenic encopresis. *Professional Psychology*, 1975, *6*, 453-456.

Yates, A. J. *Behavior therapy*. New York: John Wiley, 1970.

Young, G. C. Conditioning treatment of enuresis. *Developmental Medicine and Child Neurology*, 1965, *7*, 557-562.

Young, G. C. The treatment of childhood encopresis by conditioned gastroileal reflex training. *Behaviour Research and Therapy*, 1973, *11*, 449-503.

DRY-BED TRAINING: RAPID ELIMINATION OF CHILDHOOD ENURESIS

N. H. Azrin
T. J. Sneed
R. M. Foxx

Summary—Enuresis has been treated with moderate effectiveness by the urine-alarm method which requires many weeks of training. The present procedure used a urine-alarm apparatus but added such features as training in inhibiting urination, positive reinforcement for correct urinations, training in rapid awakening, increased fluid intake, increased social motivation to be nonenuretic, self-correction of accidents, and practice in toileting. After one all-night training session, the 24 enuretic children averaged only two bedwettings before achieving fourteen consecutive dry nights and had no major relapses. Little or no reduction in bedwetting occurred within the first two weeks for matched-control enuretics who were given the standard urine-alarm training. The results of a control-procedure showed that the new procedure did not involve Pavlovian conditioning. The new method appears to be a more rapid, effective and different type of treatment for enuresis.

About 10 per cent of all children are enuretic at the age of 6 yr. and some are still enuretic as teenagers. When enuresis is eliminated, the child's emotional adjustment has been found to be improved (Lovibond, 1964). The most effective treatment for enuresis is the urine-alarm technique which was

Reprinted from *Behaviour Research & Therapy*, 1974, *12*, 147-156. Copyright 1974 by Pergamon Press. Reprinted by permission.

The research was supported by the Illinois Department of Mental Health. We wish to thank Afton Jarvis and Dorothy Millard for serving as trainers. Reprints may be obtained from any of the authors at the Behaviour Research Laboratory, Anna State Hospital, 1000 North Main Street, Anna, Illinois 62906.

first used extensively by Mowrer and Mowrer (1938) based on their Pavlovian conditioning analysis. A loud buzzer (UCS) sounds as soon as a specially constructed bed pad is moistened by urine. The procedure requires several weeks or months, has a relatively high relapse rate, but is initially effective for as many as 80-90 per cent of enuretics (see reviews by Lovibond, 1964; Jones, 1960, Yates, 1970).

Very recently, a new procedure, the Dry-Bed procedure, has been developed from an operant model rather than a respondent model and has been used with profoundly retarded adult enuretics who were institutionalized (Azrin, Sneed and Foxx, 1973). This Dry-Bed procedure required only one night of intensive training followed by use of the urine-alarm apparatus for as little as one week. Some of the major features of the intensive training procedure were (1) large fluid intake to increase the desire to urinate, (2) hourly awakenings, (3) teaching the client to awaken to mild prompts, (4) practice in going to the toilet, (5) reinforcement for urinating in the toilet at night, (6) use of the urine-alarm apparatus to signal a bedwetting, and (7) training in awareness of the dry vs. wet condition of the bed. When an accident occurred, the client received verbal disapproval, he was required to change the bed sheets, and he was required to practice arising from the bed to walk to the toilet. After one night of intensive training, the urine-alarm apparatus remained on the bed until one week elapsed without an accident. During that time, accidents received the same treatment, but the other procedures were omitted. Bedwetting virtually ceased within only 2 or 3 days after the intensive training.

The surprisingly rapid success of the Dry-Bed procedure with the retarded adults led the authors to believe that even greater success might be achieved with non-retarded enuretic children (Azrin et al., 1973). Surprisingly, preliminary results indicated greater difficulty with the normal children. One plausible reason was that the adults had already achieved some degree of control as evidenced by their wetting their beds only 50 per cent of the time rather than the typical 100 per cent for the normal enuretic child. A second apparent reason was that the sleeping parent did not react to a signalled bed-wetting as reliably as did the night-duty attendants for the retarded residents in the institution. The procedure was, therefore, modified. To ensure the awakening of the parent, a buzzer was located in the parent's bedroom in addition to the usual buzzer in the enuretic's bedroom. Other procedural changes were made to capitalize on the greater understanding and co-operation of the non-retarded child. The child was given lengthy verbal instruction and explanations regarding the procedure, he was required to answer questions about the procedure, he was taught to engage in the required practice trials with a minimum of supervision and he was given training in deliberately delaying his urination similar to that used by Kimmel and Kimmel (1970). A second change that was natural to the home, rather than the institutional situation, was for the parent to require the child to toilet himself at the time that the parent went to sleep for the night, thereby easing the child's problem of inhibiting his urine throughout the remainder of the night.

The Dry-Bed procedure and its present modifications were devised with the view that the elimination of bedwetting was an operant process rather than Pavlovian conditioning. To evaluate this view, the present study included a procedure in which the unconditioned stimulus, the buzzer, was not present in the child's room, but only in the parent's bedroom. If the treatment process depended on Pavlovian conditioning, this omission of the UCS buzzer for the child should not result in conditioning since the remoteness of the parent's bedroom rendered the sound of the buzzer faint, if at all audible to the sleeping child. Conversely, if bedwetting did cease when the UCS buzzer was omitted, Pavlovian conditioning could not be responsible for the decrease.

METHOD

Subjects

Twenty-six children were obtained as clients in response to a newspaper advertisement that offered free treatment for bedwetters 3 yr of age or older. The only two children excluded were one who had a suspected medical problem, and one whose father did not desire a training effort. The average age was 8 yr, including three children under 6 yr of age. Nineteen were boys and seven were girls. All but one child, IQ of 70, had apparently normal intelligence. All but two had been wetting every night since infancy. Even these two exceptions had been fairly consistent bedwetters during the previous year, and prior to that time they had never remained dry for more than two months. Virtually all of the parents had sought medical assistance, and two had enrolled their children in a commercial training program with limited success.

Experimental Design

The experimental design, as outlined in Table 10.1, provided a within-subject as well as a between-subjects comparison between the standard urine-alarm method and the new Dry-Bed procedure. The 26 children were divided into 13 pairs matched for age, sex and frequency of bedwetting. Within each pair, the children were randomly assigned by a coin flip to the Control Group (Standard Urine-Alarm Procedure) or the Experimental Group (Dry-Bed Procedure). The first seven pairs were in Experiment I, whereas the subsequent six pairs were in Experiment II. The two Experimental Groups and the two Control Groups were very comparable to each other with respect to age (7.5 ± 0.5 yrs), to sex (about a 2:1 ratio of boys to girls) and to mean frequency of bedwetting (95 ± 5 per cent of the time). The Dry-Bed procedure was used in both Experiment I and II. In Experiment I, the urine-alarm sounded in the parents' bedroom as well as in the child's room, thereby providing the additional likelihood of awakening the parent (see Table 10.1). In the Dry-Bed procedure of Experiment II, the urine-alarm sounded only in the parents' room and not in the child's room, thereby providing an evaluation of the Pavlovian interpretation which requires the use of the alarm to condition the child. The within-subjects comparison was provided (see Table 10.1) by instituting the Dry-Bed procedure for the children in the control group after two weeks of training by the standard urine-alarm procedure.

Apparatus

The urine-alarm apparatus was a commonly used and commercially available bed pad (Montgomery Ward, catalog No. 53A21530). It consisted of two aluminum foil sheets connected to a battery and separated by a sheet of absorbent cloth. When the child urinated, the urine passed through the perforations of the upper sheet of aluminum foil and was absorbed by the cloth, thereby causing a small electrical current to flow between the metal sheets and triggering the buzzer in the circuit box that was connected by wires to the metal sheets. In its usual application, the buzzer was located within 6 ft of the child's bed (Child-Only Alarm Procedure). For the Dry-Bed procedure of Experiment I, a second buzzer was added that was located in the parents' bedroom such that bedwetting caused both buzzers to sound simultaneously (Parent-and-Child Alarm Procedure). For the Dry-Bed procedure of Experiment II, the buzzer sounded only in the parents' bedroom and not in the child's room (Parent-Only Alarm Procedure).

TABLE 10.1. Experimental design

	1st two weeks	*After 1st two weeks*
Exp. I Experimental Group:	Dry-Bed Procedure (Parent-and-Child Alarm)	Dry-Bed Procedure (Parent-and-Child Alarm)
Control Group:	Standard Conditioning Procedure (Child-Only Alarm)	Dry-Bed Procedure (Parent-and-Child Alarm)
Exp. II Experimental Group:	Dry-Bed Procedure (Parent-Only Alarm)	Dry-Bed Procedure (Parent-Only Alarm)
Control Group:	Standard Conditioning Procedure (Child-Only Alarm)	Dry-Bed Procedure (Parent-Only Alarm)

Control Group (Standard Urine-Alarm Procedure)

The children in the control group received training as described in the written instructions of the commercially available urine-alarm apparatus. The procedure incorporated the principal features of the standard urine-alarm conditioning method used in previously reported applications. Before the enuretic child went to bed, he was told by his parents that they were displeased with his bedwetting. The urine-alarm was placed in the bed such that when the child wet his bed, a loud alarm sounded in the circuit box located near the child's bed. The parent awakened the child, if he had not already been awakened by the alarm, and sent him to the toilet to finish urination. The parent then required the child to wash his face to assure complete awakening. The parent reset the alarm, changed the wet sheets and returned the child to bed. During the next 2 weeks, the parents reacted to bedwettings in this same manner, the urine-alarm remaining on the bed during the 2-week period. On the first night, a trainer was present throughout the night (just as he was for the children in the Dry-Bed group), to explain the procedure to the parents and to assure that they followed the standard procedure in the event of a bedwetting.

Dry-Bed Procedure

Table 10.2 outlines the sequences of procedural steps in the Dry-Bed Procedure.

The training night. About an hour before bedtime, the parents and the child were given a complete description of the Dry-Bed procedure, and the rationale for each step, as well as a review of the advantages that would result from eliminating the bedwetting problem. In order to increase the frequency of urination, the child was then given a glass of his favorite drink, and the urine-alarm was placed on his bed. The child next performed the Positive Practice procedure, which was designed to establish in the child the habit of rousing and toileting himself. The child lay in bed with the lights off and slowly and silently counted to 50 (younger children counted to a lower number) at which time he arose, walked to the toilet and attempted to urinate. Then he returned to bed where he began counting again repeating the procedure until 20 such trips were made. The parent remained outside of the room and counted the trips.

Then the child again drank as much as he could of his favorite drink, and he stated his understanding of the procedures to be followed that night, namely that he would be awakened hourly to practice going to the toilet rapidly and that, if he had an accident, he would change his bed sheets and practice toileting several times. The child then went to sleep.

Hourly awakenings. Every hour, the trainer awakened the child by using a minimal prompt needed for awakening. Occasionally the child could only be aroused by guiding him to a sitting position and gently shaking him. This guidance was faded out as soon as possible to a mere touch. Rarely, the bedroom light was turned on to assist in awakening the child. If, upon awakening, the child did not immediately walk to the bathroom, the trainer would first point toward the bathroom and then ask the child, "What did you promise to do when I woke you?" If the child still showed no signs of arising and walking to the bathroom, the trainer quickly guided him into the bathroom saying, "You have to *hurry* to the bathroom if you don't want to wet your bed!"

At the bathroom door, the trainer stopped the child and inquired whether he could inhibit urination for another hour. If the child replied that he could, the trainer praised him for his bladder control, and the child returned to bed. If the child answered that he could not inhibit urination for an hour, the trainer tried to persuade him to inhibit urination for just a few minutes, after which he praised the child for his control and allowed him to urinate. Immediately following urination, the child was praised for correct toileting and returned to bed.

When the child arrived at his bed, he was directed to feel his sheets and was asked if they were dry. He was then praised for having kept his sheets dry and encouraged to keep them dry during the next hour. Finally, the child was asked to repeat his instructions for the next hourly toileting, was given another drink, and then was allowed to return to sleep.

Accidents during training. Whenever a bedwetting accident occurred, the urine-alarm sounded. The trainer immediately disconnected the alarm, awakened the child (if he was not already awake) and reprimanded him for having wet. The child was then directed to the bathroom to finish urination. When he returned to the bedroom, he was given Cleanliness Training which required him to change his pajamas, remove the wet sheets from the bed, wipe off the mattress, and deposit the soiled linen in the appropriate place. While the child transported the soiled linen, the trainer replaced the cloth material between the metal pads of the urine-alarm apparatus and reset the device. When the bedwetter returned, he was required to obtain clean sheets and to remake his bed. After the bed sheets were changed, the child was informed that his accident indicated that he needed more practice in correct toileting in order to stay dry in the future. He was then given Positive Practice training in arising and toileting correctly until he had performed 20 practice trips to the bathroom. No re-inforcement was given for correct urination during Positive Practice. The child then returned to bed.

On the evening *following* a bedwetting accident, the child was given 20 Positive Practice trials before he retired to bed.

Post-Training Supervision

Following the single evening of intensive training, the alarm was placed on the bed each night prior to the child's bedtime. If the child has had an accident during the previous night, he was given Positive Practice before going to bed. Immediately before the patients' bedtime, usually about 11:00-12:00

TABLE 10.2.: Dry-Bed procedure

I. Intensive training (one night)
  (A) One hour before bedtime
   1. Child informed of all phases of training procedure
   2. Alarm placed on bed
   3. Positive practice in toileting (20 practice trials)
     (a) child lies down in bed
     (b) child counts to 50
     (c) child arises and attempts to urinate in toilet
     (d) child returns to bed
     (e) steps (a), (b), (c), and (d) repeated 20 times
  (B) At bedtime
   1. Child drinks fluids
   2. Child repeats training instructions to trainer
   3. Child retires for the night
  (C) Hourly awakenings
   1. Minimal prompt used to awaken child
   2. Child walks to bathroom
   3. At bathroom door (before urination), child is asked to inhibit urination for one hour (omit for children under 6)
     (a) if child could not inhibit urination
       (i) child urinates in toilet
       (ii) trainer praises child for correct toileting
       (iii) child returns to bed
     (b) if child indicated that he could inhibit urination for one hour
       (i) trainer praises child for his urinary control
       (ii) child returns to bed
   4. At bedside, the child feels the bed sheets and comments on their dryness
   5. Trainer praises child for having a dry bed
   6. Child is given fluids to drink
   7. Child returns to sleep
  (D) When an accident occurred
   1. Trainer disconnects alarm
   2. Trainer awakens child and reprimands him for wetting
   3. Trainer directs child to bathroom to finish urinating
   4. Child is given Cleanliness Training
     (a) child is required to change night clothes
     (b) child is required to remove wet bed sheet and place it with dirty laundry
     (c) trainer reactivates alarm
     (d) child obtains clean sheets and remakes bed
   5. Positive Practice in correct toileting (20 practice trials) performed immediately after the Cleanliness Training
   6. Positive Practice in correct toileting (20 practice trials) performed the following evening before bedtime

(continued)

200 / PEDIATRIC BEHAVIORAL MEDICINE

TABLE 10.2, continued

II. Post training supervision (begins the night after training)
   (A) Before bedtime
      1. Alarm is placed on bed
      2. Positive Practice given (if an accident occurred the previous night)
      3. Child is reminded of need to remain dry and of the need for Cleanliness Training and Positive Practice if wetting occurred
      4. Child is asked to repeat the parent's instructions
   (B) Night-time toileting
      1. At parents' bedtime, they awaken child and send him to toilet
      2. After each dry night, parent awakens child 30 minutes earlier than on previous night
      3. Awakening discontinued when they are scheduled to occur within one hour of child's bedtime
   (C) When accidents occurred, child receives Cleanliness Training and Positive Practice immediately upon wetting and at bedtime the next day
   (D) After a dry night
      1. Both parents praise child for not wetting his bed
      2. Parents praise child at least 5 times during the day
      3. Child's favorite relatives are encouraged to praise him

III. Normal routine initiated after 7 consecutive dry nights
   (A) Urine-Alarm is no longer placed on bed
   (B) Parents inspect child's bed each morning
      1. If bed is wet, child receives Cleanliness Training immediately and Positive Practice the following evening
      2. If bed is dry, child receives praise for keeping his bed dry
   (C) If two accidents occur within a week, the Post-Training Supervision is reinstated

---

p.m., the parents awakened their child and sent him to the bathroom. After each dry night, the parents awakened the child for toileting a half-hour earlier on the following evening. This night-time awakening was discontinued when the time of awakening was scheduled to follow the child's bedtime by no more than one hour. If a bedwetting accident occurred, the child was given the same procedure as during the initial training, namely he was awakened, reprimanded for wetting, and given Cleanliness Training and Positive Practice in toileting. Encouraging fluid intake and awakening the child hourly were discontinued during the Post-Training Supervision. The Post-Training Supervision continued until the child had been dry for 7 consecutive days.

After a dry night. If no bedwetting occurred during a given night, the next day the child was praised for having kept his bed dry. The parents were instructed to continue praising the child at appropriate and convenient times during the day, e.g., at meals and before bedtime. Close relatives or other persons whom the child admired and respected were invited to call and congratulate the child for not wetting his bed and to encourage him to remain dry at night.

Normal Routine

After the Post-Training Supervision was discontinued, the urine-alarm was no longer used nor were the nighttime awakenings continued. The parents inspected the child's bed in the morning. If the bed was wet, they required the child to remake it immediately and, before bedtime that evening, the bedwetter was given Positive Practice in correct toileting. If bedwetting occurred on 2 nights within a week, the Post-Training Supervision procedure was reinstated until the child had no accidents on seven consecutive nights.

The rationale and general description of particular procedures such as Cleanliness Training, Positive Practice, fading prompts, encouraging fluid intake, and Graduated Guidance can be found in previous reports (Azrin and Foxx, 1971; Azrin et al., 1973; Azrin, Kaplan and Foxx, 1973; Foxx and Azrin, 1972; Foxx and Azrin, 1973a; 1973b; 1973c). These procedures as used in both daytime and nighttime toilet training are described in especially great detail for use with retarded persons in Foxx and Azrin (1973a) and for normal children in Azrin and Foxx (1974).

RESULTS

Figure 10.1 shows the median number of accidents per week for the 26 enuretic children. Before training, bedwetting occurred every night. The standard urine-alarm procedure reduced the accidents slightly to six bed-wettings during the first week of training and to five accidents per week during the second week. After the one night of intensive training by the Dry-Bed procedure, the median number of accidents was only one during the first week, one during the second week, and none after the third week for the six-month follow-up. A statistical comparison of the two procedures during the first two weeks by the t test for differences showed that the number of accidents was significantly less for the children trained by the Dry-Bed procedure than by the standard urine-alarm procedure ($p < 0.005$).

Examination of the individual children trained by the standard urine-alarm procedure showed that only two of the 13 children remained dry for more than 6 nights during the first 2 weeks of training. No attempt was made to retrain these two children by the Dry-Bed procedure. The other 11 children were retrained by the Dry-Bed procedure and are included in the data points of Figure 10.1.

Examination of the individual children trained by the Dry-Bed procedure, including the 11 children who had been given the standard urine-alarm training, showed that all 24 children were trained. Figure 10.2 shows that the slowest learner had nine accidents before achieving 14 consecutive dry nights, whereas the average child (median) had only two accidents. The fastest learners had no accidents and included three of the 24 children (12 percent).

The number of accidents was virtually the same during the Parent-Only-Alarm procedure of Experiment II and the Parent-and-Child Alarm procedure of Experiment I. The mean number of accidents during the first 2 weeks was 2.6 and 2.2 respectively for the two procedures and was not significantly different.

None of the children relapsed to their pre-training level of bedwetting at any time during the six-month follow-up. The procedure had required the reinstatement of the urine-alarm apparatus should two accidents occur within a week. In only seven instances did two such accidents occur. In each instance, the child had no further accidents during the week after the urine-alarm was reinstated, and the apparatus was, therefore, again discontinued.

FIGURE 10.1.   The median number of nights per week that the 26 enuretic children wet their beds

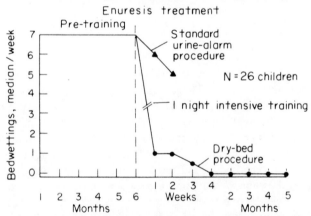

Note: The pre-training data was the report of the parent of the average number of bedwettings during the previous 6 months. The data points are presented for each week for the first 4 weeks after training and for each month thereafter. The "break" in the curve represents the single evening during which the Dry-Bed training procedure was used. The "Triangle" data points are for the 13 matched-control children who were given the standard urine-alarm conditioning procedure. The "Circle" data points are for the new Dry-Bed procedure and include the 13 enuretic children in the treatment group as well as the 11 children in the control group who failed to remain dry after 2 weeks.

FIGURE 10.2. The range of individual differences in train-ability by the new Dry-Bed procedure of the 24 enuretic children

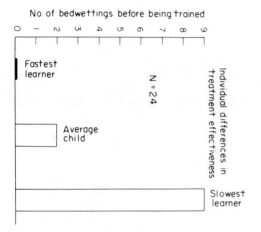

No. of bedwettings before being trained

Note: Each vertical bar designates the number of nights that the child wet his bed after the 1-night training session before he reached his criterion of 14 consecutive nights. All children were trained, the slowest child having had 9 bedwettings, the fastest children (3) having no bedwettings, and the average children (median) having two accidents before achieving the criterion of dryness.

After the intensive night of training, the urine-alarm was no longer put on the bed once the child had 7 consecutive dry nights. The criterion resulted in a median of 19 days of alarm usage after training. The Dry-Bed procedure also called for a gradual discontinuation of the nighttime awakenings. A median of 6 days was required to eliminate these awakenings.

DISCUSSION

The new procedure proved both effective and rapid in eliminating bed-wetting. Enuresis was eliminated for all 24 children without exception, including those under 6 yr of age. No major relapses occurred and no intensive retraining was necessary during the 6-month follow-up. Reinstatement of the urine-alarm apparatus for a brief one-week period was sufficient to maintain dryness in the few instances when accidents started to recur. The elimination of enuresis was almost immediate. The average child had only 2 bedwettings before achieving 2 consecutive weeks of dryness, and he wet his bed only once during the very first week after training. The training period itself was very brief; only 1 night of intensive training followed by about 2-3 weeks of the urine-alarm apparatus.

Compared with other methods of treating enuresis, the present method appears more effective and efficient. The urine-alarm conditioning procedure has been shown to be the most effective of the alternative treatments but requires months of training, permits many relapses, and does not arrest enuresis for some children (see reviews by Lovibond, 1964; Jones, 1960; and Yates, 1970). A direct comparison between the urine-alarm conditioning procedure and the new method was made in the present study by the matched-control design. The results showed the urine-alarm conditioning procedure produced only a slight reduction in bedwetting during the two-week period it was used. In contrast, the new method eliminated bedwetting almost entirely during that same period. All children who were not improved by the conditioning procedure did stop wetting when they were trained by the new Dry-Bed procedure. The new method appears to be far more rapid and effective than the urine-alarm conditioning procedure.

The present method was based on the conception of enuresis as a learning problem that involved such diverse and complex factors as motivation, degree of voluntary control over urination, parental concern, the strength of alternative responses, and the ease of arousability from sleep. The present method had used the urine-alarm apparatus for the purpose of arranging these social and motivational factors as a reaction to bedwetting. In contrast, the urine-alarm conditioning procedure has viewed enuresis as a simple problem of Pavlovian conditioning of the bladder sphincter and uses the apparatus for the purpose of associating the buzzer, as an unconditioned stimulus, with sphincter relaxation. To evaluate this conditioning function of the urine-alarm apparatus, the present method was modified (Experiment II) to omit the buzzer for the enuretic child. It was found that enuresis was eliminated just as effectively when the buzzer did not sound for the enuretic child, but only for the parent. These results demonstrate that Pavlovian conditioning did not contribute to the effectiveness of the present procedure.

One may speculate that Pavlovian-type conditioning is not the underlying process responsible for the effectiveness of the usual urine-alarm procedure. Rather, the buzzer may be merely the method of producing other and more important events such as annoyance by the child and parent at being awakened, the need to change the wet sheets, or the need to wash oneself. Other investigators also have recently challenged the role of Pavlovian conditioning in accounting for the effectiveness of the urine alarm procedure (Lovibond, 1964; Turner, Young and Rachman, 1970). Further support of this conclusion was obtained in a previous study (Azrin et. al., 1973) that found no reduction of bedwetting by the urine-alarm apparatus unless social and motivational events were associated with the buzzer.

REFERENCES

Azrin N. H. and Foxx R. M. (1971) A rapid method of toilet training the institutionalized retarded, *J. Appl. Behav. Anal. 4*, 89-99.

Azrin N. H. and Foxx R. M. (1974) *Toilet Training in Less than a Day.* Simon & Schuster, New York.

Azrin N. H., Kaplan S. J. and Foxx R. M. (1973) Autism reversal: Eliminating stereotyped self-stimulation of the retarded, *Am. J. Men. Def. 78,* 241-248.

Azrin N. H., Sneed T. J. and Foxx R. M. (1973) Dry bed: A rapid method of eliminating bedwetting (enuresis) of the retarded, *Behav. Res. & Therapy 11,* 427-434.

Foxx R. M. and Azrin N. H. (1972) Restitution: A method of eliminating aggressive-disruptive behavior of retarded and brain damaged patients. *Behav. Res. & Therapy 10,* 15-27.

Foxx R. M. and Azrin N. H. (1973a) *Toilet Training the Retarded: A Rapid Program for Days and Nighttime Independent Toileting.* Research Press, Champaign, Illinois.

Foxx R. M. and Azrin N. H. (1973b) The elimination of autistic, self-stimulatory behavior by overcorrection. *J. Appl. Behav. Anal. 6,* 1-14.

Foxx R. M. and Azrin N. H. (1973c) Dry pants: A rapid method of toilet training children. *Behav. Res. & Therapy 11,* 435-442.

Jones G. H. (1960) The behavioral treatment of enuresis nocturna. In *Behavior Therapy and the Neuroses* (Ed. Eysenck, H. J.), pp. 377-403. Pergamon Press, Oxford.

Kimmel H. D. and Kimmel E. (1970) An instrumental conditioning method for the treatment of enuresis. *J. Behav. Therapy & Exp. Psychiat. 1,* 121-123.

Lovibond S. H. (1964) *Conditioning and Enuresis.* Macmillan, New York.

Mowrer O. H. and Mowrer W. M. (1938) Enuresis—a method for its study and treatment. *Am. J. Ortho, Psychiat. 8,* 436-447.

Turner R. K., Young G. C. and Rachman S. (1970) The treatment of nocturnal enuresis by conditioning techniques, *Behav. Res. & Therapy 8,* 367-381.

Yates A. J. (1970) *Behavior Therapy,* pp. 77-106. John Wiley, New York.

HANDLING THE ENCOPRETIC CHILD

Logan Wright

Wright explores a specific symptom complex and suggests methods of intervention. Such case examples often provide insights that can be generalized to other problem areas encountered by psychologists.

At the Children's Hospital of the University of Oklahoma, we have typically seen about one child each month referred because of fecal soiling. However, after a study of this disorder was begun and the word was passed around that there was particular interest in such patients, the number of referrals increased to about one per week. Obviously, more cases of encopresis exist than is appreciated. About one half of our patients have been detected incidentally during the process of evaluating patients with more traditional psychological difficulties such as neurotic symptoms and character disorders. From our experience with encopretic patients, we have developed increased understanding of the behavioral and organic aspects of this problem and have devised a standarized treatment program that appears applicable to most cases of psychogenic encopresis.

Reprinted from *Professional Psychology*, 1973, *4*, 137-144. Copyright 1973 by the American Psychological Association. Reprinted by permission.

Logan Wright is an associate professor and chairman of the Overall Planning Committee for Human Development at the University of Oklahoma Health Sciences Center. He was formerly president of the Society for Pediatric Psychology, and is now president of APA's Division of State Psychological Association Affairs. One of his major interests is the behavioral aspects of illness. Wright also hosts a weekly television series on child rearing.

DEFINITION OF ENCOPRESIS

"Encopresis" is used to describe any voluntary or involuntary passage of feces that results in soiling of clothes. Although incidence and other normative data concerning this disorder are difficult to obtain, certain medical practitioners apparently see large number of such patients. For instance, Mercer (1967) published a report based on 138 cases. "Megacolon" is a dilation of the rectum and/or colon by retained feces. Hirschsprung's disease is the primary organic disorder that causes megacolon and encopresis. It results from an absence of ganglionic cells in the wall of the rectum or large intestine. When these nerve fibers are missing, the colon is unable to respond to the pressure created by normal amounts of fecal material with a defecation reflex. However, the incidence ratio of Hirschsprung's disease to psychogenic megacolon is quite small, in the neighborhood of 1:20 (Wright & Smith, 1971).

PATHOGENESIS

Although a few children deliberately expel feces into their clothing, soiling usually results from retention of stools. Prolonged retention produces an impacted and distended bowel. If distention persists over a prolonged period of time, loss of bowel tone and megacolon result. Bowel movements then become infrequent, with stools enlarged and painful to pass. Between movements, the anus will remain partially dilated and some seepage of fecal material onto the underclothing will occur.

Unfortunately, encopresis is a problem in which behavioral practitioners have shown very little interest. Most publications have come from pediatricians and pediatric surgeons (Davidson, 1958; Lee & Bebb, 1951; Ravitch, 1958; Sullivan, Dickinson, & Wilson, 1963). The reports of Richmond, Eddy, and Garrard (1954) and Call, Christianson, Penrose, and Backlar (1963) are representative of the very small number of studies reported in psychiatric literature. Reports by psychologists involve a few behavior modification studies. In one of these, Quarti and Renaud (1962) attempted to condition three pediatric patients by administering electroshock to the patient's spine so as to produce a defecation reflex which could then be reinforced according to operant procedures. Unpredictably, the patients' responses followed more of a classical conditioning paradigm so that the sight of the shock-producing apparatus became a conditioned stimulus (CS) which elicited the defecation without shock. In spite of the fact that 10 years have passed since this technique was first reported, no subsequent mention of it can be found. Peterson and London (1965) resorted to posthypnotic suggestion as a means of inducing their patient to defecate into a toilet so that this behavior could be reinforced. Neale (1963) and Gelber and Meyer (1965) reported on more traditional behavior therapy approaches to this problem, and Keehn (1965) provided the case history of a patient whose behavior was modified in the home setting through parent consultation. One is impressed not only with the sparse number of publications, but also with the exotic and inefficient approaches (posthypnotic suggestion, shock-producing apparatus, etc.) used to elicit defecation.

DIAGNOSTIC ASSESSMENT

In evaluating an encopretic child, certain medical as well as behavioral information must be obtained. Medical information is best obtained from a pediatrician, proctologist, or surgeon who is sophisticated in dealing with the problem. The physicians will need to indicate (a) whether the disorder has a physical etiology (e.g., Hirschsprung's disease, obstruction, etc.), (b) if the child has megacolon, (c) information concerning tone or musculature of the colon, and (d) the characteristics (large versus small, hard versus soft) of the child's stools.

If is often good to begin the psychological portion of the evaluation with an interview. Here important demographic data can be obtained, such as (a) whether the child ever achieved bowel training, (b) at what age continence was lost, (c) if toilet training had ever been coercive, (d) whether there is a history of stomach pain or other gastrointestinal (GI) problems, (e) size and viscosity of stools as observed by parents, (f) frequency and nature of soiling, (g) psychological difficulties other than soiling, (h) events that seem to coincide with or precipitate soiling, (i) reinforcement preferences that might be used to condition new behavior, and (j) family history of bowel or GI difficulties.

Intellectual development must also be assessed since it can affect encopretic symptomatology. Children of low intelligence may continue to soil at a later age because of retardation in intellectual, neurological, or physical development. Soiling can also result from less training and investment from parents who are not as responsive to their retarded child as they would be to a child who generated higher expectations. Low intelligence may also mean that the patient will be less responsive to either symptomatic or traditional psychotherapeutic treatment. An abbreviated or screening approach to intellectual evaluation is often sufficient. If the patient is found to be within the average range or above on IQ, and if the diagnostician is comfortable that there are no specific intellectual or neurological deficits, then the role of intelligence becomes less important and can for the most part be ruled out as a cause for the encopretic symptom or as a factor that might interfere with treatment. Low IQ, however, should not be regarded as a contraindication for attempting treatment. The Peabody Picture Vocabulary Test (PPVT), the Draw-A-Person Test (DAP), and the Bender-Gestalt Test are often employed for screening. More molecular measures, such as the Wechsler Intelligence Scale for Children

(WISC) or the Frostig Developmental Scale of Visual Perception, can be given if cognitive difficulties are suspected.

Psychodiagnosis of an encopretic child requires one unusual question to be answered: Do the psychogenic factors responsible for the encopresis still exist, since megacolon can perpetuate soiling long after psychogenic factors have abated? If the psychogenic factors are no longer present, then simple retraining or symptomatic treatment is indicated. However, if psychological problems persist, traditional psychotherapy should be considered along with a direct conditioning attack on the symptom.

An evaluation of the nature of any psychopathology is also important. Is the child's soiling conscious and deliberate, possibly indicating some form of character disturbance? Or is soiling the result of unconscious factors and therefore representative of a more neurotic-type disorder? The integration of psychological test data with information from medical reports is often helpful in answering this question. For example, the presence of a megacolon suggests unconscious factors to be operating while its absence suggests conscious, deliberate soiling, and thus a higher probability of character and personality disturbance. It is also important to note whether the pathology is severe, pervasive, and not limited to the encopretic symptom, or if it is circumscribed. It is not unusual to find encopretic children who remain unscathed in other areas such as affect, interpersonal behavior, task effectiveness, etc., with only the psychosomatic reaction of a few inches of intestine involved.

The question of amenability to treatment and the type of treatment indicated must also be assessed. Whether the child's parents will receive either psychotherapeutic or skill-oriented consultation or both needs to be determined. If symptomatic treatment via conditioning is indicated, an attempt should be made to evaluate what is reinforcing and therefore maintaining the soiling, and what reinforcers might be relied on in changing the patient's behavior.

A number of psychological instruments can be relied on in evaluating encopretic children. One test that has proven particularly valuable is the Rosensweig P-F Study. This test usually yields some worthwhile data concerning the child's character structure, particularly his tendency to manipulate others. The more typically used psychological techniques such as Rorschach and TAT can be relied on in the search for dynamic factors and in assaying the severity of the disturbance.

Clinical observation has suggested that encopretic children have a strong tendency to manipulate, while their mothers appear easily manipulated. For this reason, we administer locus of control scales to the child (Miller, 1963) and his parents (Bialer, 1961; Rotter, 1966). Internal locus of control for the child and external locus of control for parents are hypothesized. A Children's Problem Checklist is also completed by parents, and the number of child difficulties other than encopresis is tallied. The sheer number of problems indicated serves as a rough estimate of whether the psychopathology tends to be circumscribed or diffuse.

Psychodiagnostic information on parents usually proves helpful. For this, we administer the MMPI and a 113-item Child Rearing Attitude and Behavior Instrument, in addition to obtaining the demographic interview data mentioned earlier. Important questions concerning parents are (a) whether either parent possesses significant psychogenic characteristics, and if so their nature, (b) the amenability and receptivity of parents to treatment for themselves and/or the child, and (c) child-rearing strategies employed by parents that may be deleterious.

INTERVENTION

The initial step in the treatment program is "selling" conditioning as a powerful tool for dealing with problems that are behavioral in nature. Illustrations are given of how conditioning is employed in certain instances (such as chronic sneezing, hiccuping, vomiting, tracheotomy addiction, etc.) and how it is usually successful. The purpose is to create an expectation in the parents that what is attempted will in fact work. Positive expectations appear to be a necessary prerequisite to clinical success. A strong emphasis is also placed on the importance of compulsively following the structure of the conditioning program. It is explained that while the general principles (reward and punishment) of behavior modification are understood by most laymen, many of them obtain poor results with their reward and punishment efforts. Lack of consistency in strict adherence to the conditioning program is suggested as the reason. Parents are instructed not to allow the most minor aspect of the program to go undone. Consistency is defined as something that happens 100% of the time, and 90% consistency is regarded as no better than 10%. To help insure consistency, daily written records are required, and weekly (or more often as indicated) check-ins with the therapist by phone are also carried out.

Next, a search for reinforcers that are to be employed in the conditioning program is carried out conjointly with the parents. Treatment requires the identification of three reinforcers, two positive and one negative. Any incidence of defecation into the toilet is positively reinforced, as is going a specified period of time (usually one day) without soiling. The negative reinforcer is contingent on each incidence of soiling. Although most individuals possess highly unique reinforcement hierarchies, most encopretic children seem to respond without exception to one common source of reinforcement: the opportunity to earn time with their parents in which the child determines the nature of the activity (such as playing a game, going for a ride, watching TV, or whatever he wishes). Other positive reinforcers include tokens for the purchase of toys or candy, money, toys themselves, trips, tickets to movies or sporting events, etc. Negative reinforcers include consequences such as 30 minutes in the bathtub, loss of an opportunity to play outside after school, extra household chores, etc.

The third task of successful treatment is to insure that the child will defecate daily into the stool. This will provide the behavior that needs to be reinforced. It also avoids impaction of the colon, thus permitting it to contract toward normal size and muscle tone.

Parents are instructed to tell the child that he may try to defecate on arising in the morning. If he cannot, he is given suppositories (no prescription needed) and allowed to eat his breakfast. By the time breakfast is over, the child will need to defecate. In the event that the child does not defecate with the aid of suppositories, he is given an enema before going to school. The absolute guarantee of defecation at a predictable time (early in the morning) is considered essential to the program.

It seems regrettable that in medical literature a number of articles (e.g., Call, Christianson, Penrose, & Backlar, 1963; Richmond, Eddy, & Garrard, 1954) discourage the use of suppositories in treating encopresis. These writers usually base their discouragements on psychoanalytic theory and the notion that such practices tend to oversensitize patients to the anal erogenous zone and thereby interfere with psychosexual development. Our clinic observations have failed to indicate either anal preoccupation or other psychosexual difficulties resulting from the use of suppositories. The use of suppositories is especially preferred over orally administered cathartics, since the exact time at which oral medication will take affect cannot be predicted. Consequently, it could be at school or in other social situations where defecation would be inconvenient and unobservable by the program's implementors (parents). In addition, the possibility of adverse effects from oral cathartics on portions of the upper GI tract cannot be overlooked.

Considering the inefficient and logistically complex methods (post-hypnotic suggestion, shocking devices, etc.) that have been employed to obtain defecation, suppositories would seem to involve minimal risk. And considering the great physical and emotional harm that can be suffered by a child who soils himself, it is difficult to discourage any treatment that seems the most efficient in eradicating the symptom. The greater our experience with encopretic children, the more "sold" we become on the efficacy of suppositories.

Step 4 of the program is the weaning of the child from the cathartics (suppositories) after daily bowel movements are established and soiling discontinued. The major problem of treatment is found in this step. The process requires that a child go two weeks without soiling before weaning begins. If he achieves two soiling-free weeks, one day of the week is chosen and all external aids to defecation are discontinued for that day. If he remains soiling free for an additional week, another day's cathartics are discontinued. Thus if the child is able to go eight consecutive weeks without soiling, the cathartics will be discontinued completely. If soiling occurs during the weaning process, one day's cathartics are added for each soiling episode until the child is receiving cathartics every day or until he again goes a week without soiling. At this point the cathartics are removed for one day and the discontinuation process is reinstituted. If a child can function for two weeks without soiling after all cathartics are discontinued, the program is terminated and the child is administered the battery of posttests.

With approximately three-dozen cases, we have experienced only one failure to obtain control over the encopretic symptom. In this case the child's soiling was decreased by 75 to 90%, although he continued to soil occasionally. Compulsive adherence on the part of the mother to the prescribed program was never obtained and treatment was eventually discontinued. However, the patient did achieve complete bowel control approximately six months after treatment was discontinued. Regressions following completion of the prescribed treatment program run 10 to 15%. These patients are simply reentered into the program and usually respond quite well. Follow-up data for a period as long as four years are available on some patients, all of whom are currently free of soiling. We have recently treated one patient, who had not soiled for two and one-half years, but who regressed soon after the onset of adolescence. However, he was responsive to the program when it was reapplied.

BEHAVIORAL IMPLICATIONS

In spite of the fact that encopresis is a problem in which psychologists have showed limited interest, it appears rich with behavioral implications. For example, encopresis serves as a forceful reminder of the fact that psycho-pathology can be extremely circumscribed. There seems to be a prevailing bias among clinicians that psychopathology tends to be gross or pervasive. That is, if it is uncovered in one area of functioning (e.g., thought or affect) you will usually see evidence of it in other areas (e.g., affect, thought, interpersonal behavior, task effectiveness, etc.). Encopresis seems to challenge this assumption. As often as not, encopretic children appear to be free from significant psychopathology in other areas such as thought, affect, interpersonal functioning, etc. It is as though a few inches of the colon have responded drastically to a psychogenic factor while the rest of the organism remains unscathed.

A second interesting behavioral issue raised by encopresis involves the apparent discovery of a reinforcer that appears uniformly effective with all patients. Although we have treated hundreds of patients with dozens of difficulties (such as tracheotomy addiction, inappropriate consummatory responses, sleep disturbances, self-induced seizures, tics, enuresis, etc.), we have previously been impressed by the uniqueness of each child's reinforcement hierarchy. What is reinforcing to one child may be punishing to another. What is first in the reinforcement hierarchy of one child may be fifteenth in another's. However, with encopretic patients the reinforcement of "earned time" with parents does seem uniformly applicable. In retrospect, the most plausible explanation is that encopretic children use their soiling and/or retention of feces to manipulate parents. The "earned time" is a socially acceptable form of manipulating and controlling parents which is substituted for a socially unacceptable form of manipulation and control (encopresis).

A final basis for theoretical interest in encopretic behavior is that it graphically illustrates the three major justifications for treating symptoms as opposed to the "cause" of a given behavior. The three reasons that have been stated previously (Wright, 1970) are (a) the nonoccurrence of symptom substitution, (b) the fact that the symptom may create more psychological difficulties than the difficulties that caused the symptom, and (c) a symptom can persist after the psychogenic forces which produced the symptom have abated.

We have neither observed nor read of an instance of symptom substitution in cases of encopresis. However, encopresis is *definitely* in that category of symptoms that cause psychological difficulty as well as result from psychogenic factors. This symptom along with others such as enuresis, school phobia, etc., can oftentimes disrupt interpersonal relationships, elicit highly negative reactions from others, and generally interfere with functioning in such a way that the symptom itself accounts for a majority of the patient's total difficulty. Under such circumstances, when the symptom is gone, a great deal of the child's total psychological difficulty is removed. Finally, soiling is a symptom that can persist after the psychogenic forces that produced the soiling have abated. If a child, for some psychogenic reason, begins to retain feces, he will eventually become impacted and his colon distended. If megacolon results, soiling will continue, even though the child is no longer retaining feces for psychological reasons.

REFERENCES

Bialer, I. Conceptualization of success and failure in mentally retarded and normal children. *Dissertation Abstracts*, 1961, *21*, 2357.

Call, J. D., Christianson, M., Penrose, F. R., & Backlar, M. Psychogenic megacolon in three preschool boys: A study of etiology through collaborative treatment of child and parents. *American Journal of Orthopsychiatry*, 1963, *33*, 923-928.

Davidson, M. Constipation and fecal incontinence. *Pediatric Clinics of North America*, 1958, *5*, 749-757.

Gelber, H., & Meyer, V. Behavior therapy and encopresis: The complexities involved in treatment. *Behavior Research and Therapy*, 1965, *2*, 227-231.

Keehn, J. D. Brief case report: Reinforcement therapy of incontinence. *Behavior Research and Therapy*, 1965, *2*, 239.

Lee, C. M., & Bebb, K. C. Pathogenesis and clinical management of megacolon, with emphasis on the fallacy of the term "idiopathic." *Surgery*, 1951, *30*, 1026-1048.

Mercer, R. D. Constipation. *Pediatric Clinics of North America*, 1967, *14*, 175-185.

Miller, J. C. Role perception as reinforcement conditions in discrimination learning among culturally deprived and nondeprived children. Unpublished manuscript, George Peabody College for Teachers, 1963.

Neale, D. H. Behavior therapy and encopresis in children. *Behavior Research and Therapy*, 1963, *1*, 139-149.

Peterson, D. R., & London, P. A role for cognition in the behavioral treatment of a child's eliminative disturbance. In L. Ullmann & L. Krasner (Eds.), *Case studies in behavioral modification.* New York: Holt, Rinehart & Winston, 1965.

Quarti, C., & Renaud, J. Note preliminaire sur un noveau traitement des constipations par reflexe conditionale. *La Clinique*, 1962, *57*, 577-582.

Ravitch, M. M. Pseudo Hirschsprung's disease, *Annals of Surgery*, 1958, *147*, 781-795.

Richmond, J. B., Eddy, E. J., & Garrard, S. D. The syndrome of fecal soiling and megacolon. *American Journal of Orthopsychiatry*, 1954, *24*, 391-401.

Rotter, J. Generalized expectancies for internal vs. external control of reinforcement. *Psychological Monograph*, 1966, *80* (1, Whole No. 609).

Sullivan, D. B., Dickinson, D. D., & Wilson, J. L. The conservative management of fecal incontinence in children. *Journal of American Medical Association*, 1963, *185*, 664-666.

Wright, L. Symptoms: Is treatment mistreatment? *The Clinical Psychologist*, 1970, *23*, 6-9.

Wright, L., & Smith, E. I. The psychological management of the patient with acquired megacolon. Paper presented at the annual meeting of the American Pediatric Surgical Association, Hamilton, Bermuda, April 1971.

THERAPY OF CHRONIC CONSTIPATION IN A YOUNG CHILD BY REARRANGING SOCIAL CONTINGENCIES

H. Lal

O. R. Lindsley

HISTORY

The patient was a 3-yr-old boy, one of the two sons of East Indian parents. The father was a professor in a Canadian university and the mother a house wife.

A few days after his birth he developed severe diarrhea which resulted in hospitalization and nearly 3 months of medical treatment. After diarrhea was alleviated, he developed constipation during the next 3 yr and rarely passed a stool without a drug. During that time the patient visited the pediatrician regularly, underwent medical diagnosis several times, and received frequent pharmacological treatments.

DIAGNOSIS

At the time the boy was brought to our attention, his parents were following an elaborate daily routine in their attempt to produce stool elimina-

Reprinted from *Behavior Research and Therapy*, 1968, 6, 484-485, Copyright 1968 by Pergamon Press, Inc. Reprinted by permission.

H. Lal is presently in the Department of Phamacology at the University of Rhode Island in Kingston. O. R. Lindsley is in the School of Education at the University of Kansas in Lawrence.

The authors wish to thank Wayne Sailor for presenting the initial instructions to the mother, who found it hard to believe the senior author's earlier remedial suggestions. Visiting Wayne in his "expert's office" possibly added status—and certainly a second source—to these "ridiculously simple therapeutic suggestions which couldn't possibly work." But, of course, they did!

This study was supported by a grant (NB-05362-06) from the National Institute of Neurological Disease and Blindness, U.S. Public Health Service.

tion. The child was placed on the toilet seat for 1 or 2 hr. Mother and sometimes both parents pleaded with him to pass stools and "entertained" him during this period. If he tried to leave the seat or cried, more "affection" was emitted to "soothe him." At the end of this ritual the child was tired and was put to bed with various acts of "affection." Often the mother would lie down on the bed with the boy until he fell asleep.

A medicated suppository was administered once a week, 1 1/2-2 hr before placing the boy on the toilet seat. Invariably he defecated on the day of medication, but never without it. Occasionally defecation also took place on the following day.

The above history suggested to us that the social consequences presented to the boy by the parents for sitting on the toilet were maintaining his constipation. We therefore decided to withdraw the social events which were usually paired with sitting on the toilet, and present them as consequences for stool elimination. In order to expedite further the therapy, additional events which may accelerate the stool elimination were also sought. According to the mother, the boy liked to play in the bathtub. Therefore, playing in the tub was made contingent upon his stool elimination and programmed immediately after each bowel movement.

BEHAVIORAL MODIFICATION

In addition to the history given by the mother, a 13 days' record of ongoing toilet habits was obtained before introducing the behavioral modification program. During this phase the mother placed the boy on the toilet every day, and pleaded with him to pass stools for nearly 2 hr. At the end of this period the child was often found crying. The mother hugged the child until he calmed down and then put him to bed. The medicated suppository was administered twice during this period to elicit defecation. The data graphed in Figure 10.3 show that the stool elimination resulted only after the medication in this phase. Ten days in which no suppository was administered did not produce any defecation. The first suppository produced a bowel movement on the day of administration and also on the following day. The second suppository produced three bowel movements on the same day.

During the behavioral modification phase, the mother placed the child on the toilet seat, which was located next to a bathtub. The tub was filled with water and a few toys were placed in the tub. She told him that as soon as he had passed stools, he could call her and that she would place him in the tub for as long as he wanted. She then left the room and closed the doors. When the boy called his mother, she would come in and go directly to look into the toilet. If feces were found, she smiled, hugged and kissed the child, praised him for his response, and placed him in the tub. (If feces were not found, the mother had been told to immediately leave the bathroom—but surprisingly this never happened!)

The modification phase was initiated by eliciting the first bowel movement with the medicated suppository prescribed by his physician. The presentation of social consequences followed immediately after the elicited bowel movement. The boy acquired the elimination response instantaneously, and after the first modification session did not ever require another suppository (Figure 10.3). The possibility of this change in bowel movement rate occurring by chance is three in one hundred thousand times (Fisher's exact formula applied to the Mid-median test). According to his mother, who administered the behavioral modification, he began to ask for the toilet seat himself during the latter part of this phase. Time spent on the toilet seat was not reinforcing by itself, since it was reduced gradually from nearly 2 hr in the beginning to a mere 15 min (approximately) in the end.

During the final, post-treatment phase, the mother placed him on the toilet whenever he asked for it and gave him a bath daily, but not necessarily

FIGURE 10.3. Permanent acceleration of bowel movements of a 3-yr-old boy, from none without a suppository laxative (chronic constipation) to one per day, by 2 weeks of caressing the boy immediately after each movement rather than before

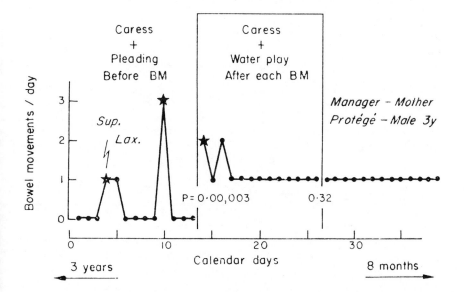

after his defecation. The boy, however, was helped from the toilet seat by his mother as he was unable to get down himself. After 14 days of the post-treatment recording, the boy returned to his home in Canada. The last communication from his parents, nearly 8 months after treatment, reported the child to be regular in his toilet habits and free from constipation. The toilet routine appeared to be maintained by its natural consequences. The transfer from the programmed social consequences to the natural home conditions occurred without any response decrement.

DISCUSSION

The social consequences which apparently maintained toilet sitting and constipation so successfully for nearly 3 yr were equally powerful in generating bowel movements when the contingencies of their presentation were rearranged. Making the parental caresses contingent upon bowel movements rather than toilet sitting, successfully accelerated bowel movements and at the same time decreased the duration of toilet sitting.

This case history provides still another example of maladaptive child behavior being maintained by social consequences unwittingly presented by the parents. Our case report also provides another instance in which a symptom, traditionally thought to be a disorder requiring medical attention (but resisting all traditional medical treatment!), was actually a learned response and was immediately responsive to behavior therapy by merely rearranging social contingencies.

11

EATING

INTRODUCTION

Feeding

In the normal course of development, a child must progress from parent feeding to self-feeding, and from "baby" foods to adult foods. Children often refuse to make these transitions. The incidence of feeding problems in young children may be as high as 45 percent (Bentovim, 1970). The child may respond to parental urgings with tantrums or refusal to eat; and these reactions may effectively control the parent's behavior so that the child's habits are allowed to continue, sometimes at the expense of good nutrition. The eating problem may be reinforced by the attention given by the parent during eating episodes. If the child has had a gastrointestinal problem requiring a special diet, which is associated with extra maternal attention, a return to the normal diet may be resisted. A child may also expect new foods to be distasteful. Such expectations lead to food refusal, and are reinforced by attention and successful avoidance of unwanted food. Traditional therapy techniques have included forced feeding by parents, which may result in gagging or swallowing foods whole; withholding all inappropriate food until hunger causes appropriate eating; or verbal and physical threats. Rarely are these effective.

The behavioral approach to eating problems recognizes the reinforcing potential of parental attention and successful food avoidance. However, simple withholding of attention and withdrawal from all inappropriate food may not result in appropriate eating behavior. Children may cry and starve themselves until the parents yield to their demands (Bernal, 1972). In one study (Thompson & Linscheid, 1976) a two-and-a-half-year-old boy refused to eat anything but puréed baby food, and the mother always gave in to the child's demands after her attempts resulted in tantrums. The therapist shaped the child's eating by reinforcing appropriate eating behavior with praise, attention, and a favorite cookie; noncooperation was ignored. Gradually, the child was required to eat more appropriate food to get his cookie. The mother was trained in these techniques, and also learned not to use verbal or physical threats. After nine sessions the child was eating adequately.

Behavioral techniques have also been used with older children who for medical reasons must exercise special dietary control. Magrab and Papadopoulou (1977) used a system of token reinforcement to change the eating and drinking habits of children on hemodialysis for whom dietary instructions, increased staff attention, parent counseling, and medical consultation had all been unsuccessful.

In a study by Bernal (1972), a nine-year-old girl who would not feed herself adequately and who refused table foods was treated by a gradual shaping process. The parents were trained in techniques that involved the use of social and food reinforcers for appropriate eating. The gradual nature of this approach is important for keeping trauma to the child and the parents at a minimum. The study emphasizes the importance of monitoring the parent's behavior, since many mothers are susceptible to their child's control techniques, such as tantrums, and may interrupt appropriate shaping techniques when tantrums occur. The study by Palmer, Thompson, and Linschied (1975) included here likewise shaped inappropriate eating using social attention and preferred foods as reinforcers. This report illustrates how a careful behavioral analysis of the mother-child interaction during feeding showed that the child's continuous questioning and the mother's answers interfered with eating. Since this interaction appeared rewarding, social attention was tried successfully as a reinforcer.

Pica

Pica is the ingestion of nonfood objects such as dirt, bugs, soap, or paint chips. In psychotic children, the behavior may persist (Bakwin & Bakwin, 1972), but in normal children pica usually begins around age two and disappears by the fourth or fifth year (Kessler, 1966). The incidence of pica seems to be higher in homes where the physical environment is inadequate in stimulation or maternal attention, such as those of lower socioeconomic families (Kessler, 1966). According to Woody (1971), whose paper follows in this chapter, the etiology of pica is still unknown. Some therapists believe that the child may be compensating for a nutritional deficit, or have some unfulfilled oral needs, but neither of these theories has led to any effective therapy. The behavioral approach discussed by Woody is based partly on the possibility that pica provokes reactions from parents that are rewarding in the sense of providing attention.

Given the usual age of occurrence for this disorder, contingent withdrawal of social attention after pica, together with increased attention after periods of no pica, would be indicated. The increased attention from the mother would also be a step in correcting a possibly inadequate mother-child relationship, a factor cited as contributory by psychodynamic theorists.

References

Alford, G. S., Blanchard, E. B., & Buckley, T. M. Treatment of hysterical vomiting by modification of social contingencies: A case study. *Journal of Behavior Therapy and Experimental Psychiatry*, 1972, *3*, 209-212.

Bakwin, H., & Bakwin, R. M. *Behavior disorders in children* (3rd ed.). Philadelphia: Saunders, 1972.

Bentovim, A. The clinical approach to feeding disorders of childhood. *Journal of Psychosomatic Research*, 1970, *14*, 267-276.

Bernal, M. E. Behavioral treatment of a child's eating problem. *Journal of Behavior Therapy and Experimental Psychiatry*, 1972, *3*, 43-50.

Cunningham, C. E., & Linscheid, T. R. Elimination of chronic infant ruminating by electric shock. *Behavior Therapy*, 1976, *7*, 231-234.

Fullerton, D. T. Infantile rumination: A case report. *Archives of General Psychiatry*, 1963, *9*, 593-600.

Hollowell, J. G., & Gardner, L. I. Rumination and growth failure in male fraternal twins: Association with disturbed family environment. *Pediatrics*, 1965, *36*, 565-571.

Ingersoll, B., & Curry, F. Rapid treatment of persistent vomiting in a 14-year-old female by shaping and time-out. *Journal of Behavior Therapy and Experimental Psychiatry*, 1977, *8*, 305-307.

Kanner, L. *Child psychiatry* (3rd ed.). Springfield, Ill.: C. C. Thomas, 1957.

Kessler, J. W. *Psychopathology of childhood*. Englewood Cliffs, N.J.: Prentice-Hall, 1966.

Lang, P. J. Behavior therapy with a case of nervous anorexia. In L. P. Ullmann & L. Krasner (Eds.), *Case studies in behavior modification*. New York: Holt, Rinehart & Winston, 1965, 217-221.

Magrab, P. R., & Papadopoulou, Z. L. The effect of a token economy on dietary compliance for children on hemodialysis. *Journal of Applied Behavior Analysis*, 1977, *10*, 573-578.

Murray, M. E., Keele, D. K., & McCarver, J. W. Treatment of rumination with behavioral techniques: A case report. *Behavior Therapy*, 1977, *8*, 999-1003.

Palmer, S., Thompson, R. J., Jr., & Linscheid, T. R. Applied behavior analysis in the treatment of childhood feeding problems. *Developmental Medicine and Child Neurology*, 1975, *17*, 333-339.

Richmond, J. B., Eddy, E., & Green, M. Rumination: A psychosomatic syndrome of infancy. *Pediatrics*, 1958, *22*, 49-55.

Sajwaj, T., Libet, J., & Agras, S. Lemon-juice therapy: The control of life-threatening rumination in a six-month-old infant. *Journal of Applied Behavior Analysis*, 1974, *7*, 557-563.

Thompson, R. J., Jr., & Linscheid, T. R. Adult-child interaction analysis: Methodology and case application. *Child Psychiatry and Human Development*, 1976, *7*, 31-42.

Walen, S. R., Hauserman, N. M., & Lavin, P. J. *Clinical guide to behavior therapy*. Baltimore: Williams and Wilkins, 1977.

Wolf, M. M., Birnbrauer, J. S., Williams, T., & Lawler, J. A note on apparent extinction of the vomiting behavior of a retarded child. In L. P. Ullmann & L. Krasner (Eds.), *Case studies in behavior modification*. New York: Holt, Rinehart & Winston, 1965, 364-366.

Woody, R. H. Controlling pica via an environmental-psycho-behavioral strategy: With special reference to lead poisoning. *The Journal of School Health*, 1971, *41*, 548-555.

APPLIED BEHAVIOR ANALYSIS IN THE TREATMENT OF CHILDHOOD FEEDING PROBLEMS

Sushma Palmer
Robert J. Thompson Jr.
Thomas R. Linscheid

INTRODUCTION

In recent years evidence has accumulated which suggests that feeding problems in children are a significant clinical entity. Among the most frequent difficulties encountered are prolonged subsistence on pureed or "junior" foods because of neuromotor dysfunction, mechanical obstruction or mismanagement, and a variety of others such as bizarre food habits, dislike of many foods, tantrums during meals, or simply refusal to eat. Data from the Georgetown University Affiliated Program for Child Development show that 33 per cent of patients examined in the Nutrition Division between 1971 and 1973 exhibited feeding problems. Similar reports from other quarters provide further evidence that feeding problems occur frequently, particularly in the pre-school handicapped child. One child-development center reports an incidence of 13 to 33 per cent of such problems in their nutrition division population (Coffey and Crawford 1971), and a recent survey of five state institutions in the Massachusetts area noted that one in every three patients suffered from difficulty in chewing or swallowing (McKrensky 1974).

Despite growing recognition of a high incidence of feeding problems in children, a review of the literature reveals virtually no classification system, discussion of the incidence, diagnostic criteria or appropriate treatment methods. There is an obvious need for a classification of feeding problems and integration of treatment techniques.

AUTHORS' APPOINTMENTS: Sushma Palmer, director of Nutrition, Robert J. Thompson, Jr., director of Psychology, Thomas R. Linscheid, staff psychologist; University Affiliated Program for Child Development, Georgetown University Hospital, Washington, DC 20007.

A partial reason for the paucity of information may be that children with feeding problems may be referred to a variety of disciplines, each of which views the problem from its own disciplinary perspective and uses treatment methods appropriate to that discipline. Furthermore, most attention appears to be given to the treatment of feeding difficulties in specific disabilities (Clancy et al. 1969) rather than regarding them as a separate clinical entity which may be encountered in a variety of disorders and disabilities, as well as in normal children. There are many reports of the treatment of feeding problems in children with cerebral palsy or mental retardation (e.g. Adair 1960, Bosley 1966) and frequently the methods of Blanchard (1966) and Mueller (1973) are recommended by occupational and speech therapists to improve neuromotor co-ordination and promote development. Similarly, for the treatment of behavior problems related to eating, psychologists have recommended behavior modification (Edwards and Lilly 1966, Bernal 1972). For orthopedic problems which hinder feeding, suggestions include the use of special feeding apparatus (Hall 1951, Gertenrich 1970), and for multiple food dislikes the acceptable procedure traditionally has been modification in texture, variety, color and the method of preparation of food (Lowenberg 1948, Augustine et al. 1950) and, more recently, behavior modification (Ireton and Guthrie 1972).

Our own experience indicates that feeding problems seldom have a single cause and that the symptomatology typically includes behavioral, nutritional and developmental components. The clinical management of feeding problems requires an integrated interdisciplinary approach to diagnosis and treatment; it is likely that the knowledge and understanding derived from such a collaboration will help to delineate the entity of "feeding problems." We have developed an interdisciplinary approach, the essence of which is applied behavior analysis, and which incorporates behavioral, nutritional and developmental principles in the diagnosis and treatment of feeding problems. The use of applied behavior analysis for the treatment of tantrums during meals has been described previously (Thompson and Palmer 1974). This present paper reports its application to another frequent problem, prolonged subsistence on pureed foods, and suggests behavioral mismanagement as a cause.

It has been proposed that there is a critical or sensitive period for the introduction of solid foods, that missing this period creates subsequent feeding problems, and that one of the causes of this problem is "mismanagement" (Illingworth and Lister 1964). Other causes for late introduction of solids cited by those authors are dysphagia in infancy because of congenital abnormalities or neuromuscular factors; mental retardation; delayed neuromotor development; and obstructive lesions (Illingworth and Lister 1964, Illingworth 1969).

Our experience indicates that "mismanagement" (or more appropriately "behavioral mismanagement") is indeed a significant cause of such difficulties. Of the 52 cases with delayed introduction of solid foods we have examined in the last two years, 78.8 per cent were due to neuromotor dysfunction (including dysphagia in infancy and mental retardation), 3.8 per cent were due to mechanical obstructions (obstructive lesions) and 17.3 per cent seemed to be due primarily to behavioral mismanagement, defined as failure to introduce solids at the appropriate age, forced feeding, or excessive parental anxiety during meals. In addition to specific evidence of mismanagement, Illingworth (1958) maintains that mismanagement is inferred when the patient's refusal or inability to accept solids appears to be dissociated from and significantly delayed in comparison with other developmental milestones.

The following case history describes the application of behavior modification to a youngster who developed extreme dislike of solid food as a result of behavioral mismanagement.

CASE HISTORY

J. is the sixth child of a 32-year-old white mother. The parental history indicated that the mother had been severely anemic and required folic acid and iron supplements during pregnancy. J. was delivered spontaneously and weighed 5 lb 12 oz (2623g). He had a myelomeningocele which was corrected surgically on the second day of life. He remained in hospital for the first six months of life, and his developmental milestones thereafter, according to his mother, were markedly delayed.

In May 1973, at six years of age, J. was referred to the Georgetown University Affiliated Program for Child Development for assessment of his level of functioning, in order to plan appropriate treatment. He was paraplegic and generally was confined to a wheelchair. He was functioning in the borderline range of intelligence, his gross motor skills were at the six-month level, fine motor skills were below the three-year level, and receptive language was at about the 4 1/2 year level. He had a highly idiosyncratic language pattern, consisting of many stereotyped and irrelevant statements.

He weighed 27 lb (12.25kg) and was well below the third percentile for weight and height, showing severe growth retardation. Nutrient analysis of a seven-day diet record showed it to be deficient in calories, vitamin A and vitamin C, and to be excessive in iron and calcium, compared with the Recommended Dietary Allowance (RDA) for age, as well as in comparison with nutrient levels per centimetre of height using the RDA table (National Academy of Sciences 1973).

Up to six months of age J. had progressed normally to supplementing foods. However, he did not progress beyond pureed foods, despite frequent but late attempts to introduce lumpy and solid foods into his diet. His repeated refusal to eat these foods had led the parents to resort to forced feeding (holding him down and forcing food into his mouth), which frequently resulted in gagging and sometimes swallowing the food whole.

It appeared that J. had developed an extreme fear of solid foods, possibly because of the failure to introduce them at the critical period and the subsequent forced feeding. In addition, unlike most infants, J. reportedly had not mouthed objects, and this lack may have added to his apprehension about putting textured foods into his mouth.

A major component of the treatment program designed for J. was an applied behavior analysis program which was intended to overcome his refusal of solid foods, to eliminate infantile feeding habits and gradually to establish a nutritionally adequate diet.

Procedure

To establish an adequate nutritional intake, the behavioral approach employed was similar to the one described previously (Thompson and Palmer 1974). The habitual feeding patterns of J. and his family fostered the maintenance of infantile feeding behavior and his refusal of solid foods. J. did not feed himself; this was done primarily by the mother. To ascertain what behaviors needed to be altered and what effective reinforcers could be used, a videotaped baseline feeding session was conducted at the Center, the mother being instructed to keep as nearly as possible to the usual routine. Subsequent analysis of the videotape showed that J. made many irrelevant remarks (mainly questions) which effectively circumvented the task of eating. His mother contributed to the process by answering him, by posing questions herself, and by conversing with him almost constantly.

It was decided that the amount of verbal interaction must be reduced and that the variety and amount of food consumed, particularly of solid foods, must be increased. It would also be necessary to overcome his dislike of solid foods. Praise, attention, and encouragement, together with the selective presentation of preferred foods, were to be used as reinforcers.

Over a three-week period, 13 treatment sessions were conducted at the Center late in the afternoon, J. having had only a small lunch earlier in the day. All the sessions were videotaped, and several graduate students and professional staff acted as therapists by assuming the mother's role of assisting J. to eat. The mother watched the sessions on a monitor and attempted to implement the therapist's techniques when feeding J. at home. The length of each session varied, but J. was required to eat at least one spoonful of food before the session could be ended.

At the beginning of each session, a hospital tray of food was laid on a table in front of J. He was given the opportunity to eat a variety of pureed, minced and bite-sized foods, in addition to milk. The therapist placed food on the spoon and put the spoon into J's hand. Typically, he ate the pureed food and refused solids. Several times he sat for as long as an hour with minced or bitesized food on his spoon. His crying increased as he gradually brought the spoon closer to his mouth. When he had eaten the food he was praised and sometimes offered a spoonful of preferred food such as pudding. The preferred food was always coupled with praise and attention so that eventually these reinforcers could be used to maintain appropriate behavior without having to present the preferred foods. The mother's brief entry into the room was also used occasionally as a reinforcer.

When J. refused food or avoided eating by making irrelevant statements or asking inappropriate questions, the therapist stopped talking and turned away from him, and did not turn back until J. had ceased the inappropriate behavior. As soon as J. had succeeded in putting the food into his mouth, the therapist praised him and offered a preferred food. Gradually the offering of preferred foods decreased so that it occurred not after every spoonful but only after four or five.

When the treatment program ended, and during two follow-up sessions, J's mother resumed her usual role of assisting him to eat.

Results

The length of the treatment sessions ranged from 60 to 210 minutes (mean 102 minutes). Table 11.1 shows the amounts of each type of food eaten by J. during the baseline, treatment and follow-up sessions.

No food was eaten during the baseline session conducted by the mother, but by the 13th session, which she also conducted, he ate 147g of food. The change in texture of food was also noteworthy, from entirely pureed gradually to minced and then to bite-sized food from session 5 onwards. Session 5 was a turning point. Although J. had eaten a small amount of minced food during session 2, he continually refused it in session 5, while crying and pleading to be taken home. It was essential to teach J. that the session would end only when he had eaten, therefore his crying was ignored for more than three hours until he ate one spoonful of minced food, after which he was immediately taken home.

The reduced amount of food eaten during sessions 10 to 12 reflects a change from quantity to texture of foods eaten and the eating patterns having become more normal. During these sessions J. was offered only small amounts of bite-sized food on a plate rather than on a tray.

Follow-up at four months indicated that treatment gains had been sustained. Attempts to obtain similar data at 12 months follow-up were unsuccessful since J. refused to eat on that occasion. This was attributed to apprehension because of his long absence from the Center. However, data were obtained on the range and content of his diet at home over 12 months.

Table 11.2 compares the range of foods eaten by J. during a seven-day period before treatment and at four and 12 months after treatment. Not only had the texture and variety increased noticeably, but at the time of follow-up

TABLE 11.1. Type and amount (gms) of food eaten during baseline, treatment and follow-up sessions

Type of food	Baseline*	Treatment sessions													Four months Follow-up*
		1	2	3	4	5	6	7	8	9	10	11	12	13*	
Liquid	0	28	29	39	15	9	35	55	36	73	0	0	0	53	28
Pureed	0	41	50	56	58	112	113	148	41	14	24	3	12	80	†
Minced	0	0	6	0	0	3	44	30	22	53	13	0	6	0	†
Bite-sized	0	0	0	0	0	0	0	0	0	0	45	38	6	13	120
Total	0	69	86	95	73	124	192	233	98	140	81	41	24	147	148

*session conducted by mother
†not offered

228

TABLE 11.2. Foods eaten during a seven-day period before treatment and at follow-up

Baseline	Four months follow-up		12 months follow-up	
Milk	Milk	Spaghetti	Milk	Peas
Enriched oatmeal	Oatmeal	Frankfurters	Oatmeal	Frankfurters
Enriched rice cereal	Cream of wheat	Meat loaf	Cream of wheat	Roast beef
Pureed beef	Scrambled eggs	Cheese	Bread	Hamburger
Pureed turkey	Orange juice	Canned peaches	Potatoes	Macaroni cheese
Pureed green beans	Bread	Ice cream	Tomato soup	Spaghetti & meatballs
Pureed corn	Mashed potatoes		Cheese soup	Cream cheese
Butterscotch pudding	Vegetable soup		Chicken soup	Peaches
Vanilla pudding	Baked beans		Baked beans	Ice cream
Chocolate pudding	Macaroni cheese		Broccoli	Vanilla pudding

the diet appeared to be almost appropriate for age. There had also been an improvement in nutrient intake.

Before treatment, J's diet was deficient in calories and vitamins A and C, and was excessive in iron and calcium. Four months after treatment, nutrient intake over a seven-day period showed increases in caloric and vitamin A and C intake to within two-thirds of the RDA table and a substantial reduction in iron and calcium intake (Table 11.3). 12 months after treatment, all the nutrients analyzed were over 70 per cent of the RDA table; in fact, with the addition of a multivitamin and mineral supplement (recommended after the four-month follow-up), J's diet meets 100 per cent of the RDA standard for all nutrients except calories.

J's weight increased from 27 lb (12.25kg) before treatment to 27.5 lb (12.48kg) at the four-month follow-up, and to 29.75 lb (13.15kg) at the 12-month follow-up.

Discussion

The successful use of applied behavior analysis for nutritional problems requires careful planning of the total program, as well as of each individual treatment session. The problem must be analyzed in terms of what behaviors need to be altered, what at present sustains these behaviors, and what reinforcers and resources can be used to bring about the necessary changes. Specific steps in the treatment program can then be devised.

It is essential that the therapist and the parents appreciate the large amount of effort and commitment needed if the treatment is to succeed. It is not possible to predict the number of treatment sessions; and in order to sustain

TABLE 11.3. Nutrient intake as percentage of Recommended Daily intake (RDA) before treatment and at follow-up

Nutients	Baseline (% RDA)	Four months follow-up (% RDA)	12 months follow-up (% RDA)
Calories	44	67	73
Protein	93	102	110
Vitamin A	43	66	81
Vitamin C	42	75	75
Iron	500	68	70
Calcium	300	68	95

any gains achieved during treatment the family must learn the techniques found to be effective during treatment sessions and attempt to implement them at home. In the present case, this was accomplished by having the mother view the treatment sessions on a video monitor while one of the authors explained the techniques and answered her questions.

The point at which intensive therapy should be ended is determined by the therapist and the parents, and will depend on the degree to which the objectives have been met. In J.'s case, the goals of overcoming his refusal of solid foods and eliminating infantile feeding habits were met successfully. The third goal of gradually establishing a nutritionally adequate diet had been substantially achieved 12 months after treatment.

Applied behavior analysis has many advantages in the treatment of feeding problems. Since the treatment can be given on an out-patient basis, the child does not suffer any drastic environmental change. The method also allows the parents to learn the technique at first-hand through videotape monitoring and to practice it at home under professional guidance. Furthermore, the danger of dehydration or severe weight-loss is minimal, since initially the treatment takes place during one meal only. In contrast to the method described by Holser-Buehler (1973), applied behavior analysis can be modified for use in a variety of cases, rather than being one regime applicable to every child.

Our own clinical experience suggests the classification of feeding problems shown in Table 11.4. We view this merely as a preliminary attempt to delineate the types of feeding problems arising mainly from one of three causes. Although we show only three main causes, we would emphasize that the

TABLE 11.4. Classification of feeding problems

	Possible causes		
Major problems	Behavioral mismanagement	Neuromotor dysfunction	Mechanical obstruction
Meal-time tantrums	X		
Bizarre food habits	X		
Multiple food dislikes	X		
Prolonged subsistence on pureed food	X	X	X
Delay or difficulty in sucking, swallowing or chewing	X	X	X
Delay in self-feeding	X	X	X

symptomatology may be complex in each case. We expect that as interest develops in this field more categories will be added and definitions refined. In a broader sense, the recognition that feeding problems are a clinical entity might lead to the integration of the valuable work being done in may disciplines, and to such problems receiving considerably more attention than they do at present.

SUMMARY

This paper discusses behavioral mismanagement as a cause of feeding problems in children and reports the case of a six-year-old handicapped boy who was subsisting almost entirely on pureed foods at the time of his referral. Treatment with applied behavior analysis resulted in his acceptance of foods normal for his age, and at follow-up 12 months after treatment the variety of foods eaten and the nutrient intake were virtually normal for his age.

The authors discuss the frequent occurrence of feeding problems in children and their possible causes. They propose that such problems constitute a clinical entity and suggest a preliminary classification system for them.

REFERENCES

Adair, R. (1960) "Home care and feeding of a mentally retarded child." *Journal of the American Dietetic Association, 36*, 133.

Augustine, G., McKinley, M., Laughlin, S. L., James, E. L., Eppright, E. (1950) "Nutritional adequacy, cost and acceptability of lunches in an Iowa school lunch program." *Journal of the American Dietetic Association, 26*, 654.

Bernal, M. E. (1972) "Behavioral treatment of a child's eating problem." *Journal of Behavior Therapy and Experimental Psychiatry, 3*, 43.

Blanchard, I. (1966) "Developing motor control for self feeding." *Cerebral Palsy Journal, 27* (5), 9.

Bosley, E. (1966) "Teaching the cerebral palsied to chew." *Cerebral Palsy Journal, 27* (4), 8.

Clancy, H., Entsch, M., Rendle-Short, J. (1969) "Infantile autism: the correction of feeding abnormalities." *Developmental Medicine and Child Neurology, II*, 569.

Coffey, K. R., Crawford, J. (1971) "Nutritional problems commonly encountered in the developmentally handicapped." In Smith, M.A. (Ed.) *Feeding the Handicapped Child.* Memphis, Tenn.: University of Tennessee Child Developmental Center.

Edwards, M., Lilly, R. T. (1966) "Operant conditioning: an application to behavioral problems in groups." *Mental Retardation, 4* (4), 18.

Gertenrich, R. L. (1970) "A simple, adaptable drinking device for mental retardates lacking arm-hand control." *Mental Retardation* (Abstract), *8*, (3), 51.

Hall, M. E. (1951) "Two feeding appliances." *American Journal of Occupational Therapy, 5* (2), 52.

Holser-Buehler, P. (1973) "Correction of infantile feeding habits." *American Journal of Occupational Therapy, 26*, 331.

Illingworth, R. S. (1958) "Dissociation as a guide to developmental assessment." *Archives of Disease in Childhood, 33*, 118.

_____ (1969) "Sucking difficulties in infancy: diagnostic problem of dysphagia." *Archives of Disease in Children, 44*, 655.

_____ , Lister, J. (1964) "The critical or sensitive period, with special reference to certain feeding problems in infants and children." *Journal of Pediatrics, 65*, 839.

Ireton, C. L., Guthrie, H. A. (1972) "Modification of vegetable eating behavior in pre-school children." *Journal of Nutrition Education, 4* (3), 100.

Lowenberg, M. E. (1948) "Food preferences of young children." *Journal of the American Dietetic Association, 24*, 430.

McKrensky, M. (1974) "After nutrition legislation and guidelines what?" Paper presented at the 57th annual American Dietetic Association meeting. Philadelphia, Pa.

Mueller, H. (1973) "Pre-speech evaluation and therapy." Presented at the Bobath Course at Suffix Rehabilitation Center, Long Island, N.Y.

National Academy of Sciences - National Research Council (1973) *Recommended Dietary Allowances*, revised 1973. Washington, D.C.: National Academy of Sciences.

Thompson, R. J., Palmer, S. (1974) "Treatment of feeding problems: a behavioral approach." *Journal of Nutrition Education, 6* , 63.

CONTROLLOING PICA VIA
AN ENVIRONMENTAL—PSYCHOBEHAVIORAL
STRATEGY:
WITH SPECIAL REFERENCE
TO LEAD POISONING

Robert H. Woody

Pica is the behavioral habit of ingesting inedible materials, such as clay, plaster, paint, and ashes. The materials chosen may be quite varied; Verville (1) reports that Kanner's (2) pica cases used such substances as dirt, rags, splinters, ashes, plaster, match heads, shoe-strings, hair, rubber, coal, stones, toys, buttons, clothing, soap, thread, paper, sticks, bugs, feces, polish, and oilcloth. Since most infants (during the first year of life) put everything in their mouths but gradually learn to discriminate edible objects from inedible ones (usually between one and two years of age), the category of pica necessarily involves developmental considerations. Pica is clinically significant when the child purposely and persistently searches for inedible substances (as contrasted to the aimless mouthing of casually encountered inedible objects) and swallows them.

In a review and interpretation of the research on pica, Kessler (3) indicates: mothers are apparently not prone spontaneously to report pica; there seems to be a higher incidence of pica in lower socio-economic samples and in Negro samples than in white samples (even when economic factors are controlled); slightly more boys than girls develop pica (but this may be a false finding, in that it is derived from mental hygiene data and it is well established that boys are more apt than girls to be referred to such a clinic); there is no significant correlation between pica and intelligence; a little over 20% of the children referred to a mental hygiene clinic, upon questioning, were found to have pica and other studies revealed as high as 35% (for a Negro sample). Kessler

Reprinted from *Journal of School Health,* 1971, *41,* 548-555. Copyright 1971 by the American School Health Association. Reprinted by permission.

Robert H. Woody is professor of psychology at the University of Nebraska at Omaha.

concludes that the studies "show a surprisingly high prevalence of pica, especially in clinic patients" (p. 107); she points out that pica is usually established during the second year of life and disappears by the fourth or fifth year, but that "there are some school children who persist in licking, chewing, or swallowing lead pencils, backs of chairs, and so on" (p. 107).

There are two basic theories for the etiology of pica. One position maintains that the child has some sort of specific nutritional deficit and is literally searching for compensation via his indiscriminate ingestion of inedible substances. The other position asserts that pica is primarily due to psychological factors; that is, that the child has an unmet oral need or exaggerated orality, probably connected to the inadequacy of his affective relationship with his mother.

Physical and cultural conditions within the child's environment appear to have a relationship to the development of pica. Specifically, there seems to be a higher incidence of pica in children from lower socio-economic backgrounds. Kessler (3) states:

> An inadequate physical environment seems to play a causative role in many cases. A child who is bored, restless, cooped up, and unsupervised and who has few toys or little planned activity, may well begin to chew the furniture or window sills. But some children develop pica even when they have good food, interesting and safe toys, and conscientious parents. Such children may be choosing to do this as a way of defying their mothers' edicts. Persistent pica of this type may be an early sign of emotional disturbance, worthy of attention and intervention quite aside from the attendant physical dangers. (p. 108)

It is important to note that while there are strong indications of a relationship between pica and factors within the physical environment and that pica appears to have a significant statistical correlation with several cultural and socio-economic conditions, *the true etiology of pica has yet to be determined.*

The possibility of lead poisoning is a major hazard for pica children. Ingesting particles from an object or a surface covered with a lead-based paint is one of the most common means by which children elevate their blood-lead level. This usually occurs in older homes, where painting was done prior to 1940 (at which time efforts were made to eliminate lead from paints), and particularly in those houses that are in disrepair. Crude estimates reveal that there are approximately 80 million houses in the United States built before 1940, about 7.5 million of which are in distinct disrepair. For children living in such houses there exists the real possibility of lead poisoning.

The alarming fact is that most environmental health specialists accept that the pica child with lead poisoning cannot be treated *per se*, but that rather the emphasis should be on renovating older houses. It has been asserted that the approximate average of $1,200 to $1,500 spent for renovations is a small price to pay (and this is probably a conservative cost estimate), especially when the alternatives are the death of the child or the expensive practice of institutionalizing a child who has suffered severe brain damage as a result of lead poisoning.

The foregoing environmental renovation practice is labeled "alarming" because, contrary to the popular professional misconception, it is quite feasible to alter the pica behavioral habits. The techniques for accomplishing this behavioral change are derived from behavioristic psychology. This paper will provide an overview of the technical methodology.

BEHAVIORAL MODIFICATION TECHNIQUES FOR PICA

Behavioral modification techniques are rooted in learning theory. It is accepted that behavior is learned; that is, when reinforcements occur in conjunction with a particular behavioral act, that act tends subsequently to occur more readily because of having been reinforced. Thus behavioral problems are viewed simply as maladaptive habits; the psychodynamic theory that behavioral problems represent emotional conflicts that must be resolved by insight oriented techniques (e.g., psychoanalytically oriented psychotherapy) is refuted by behavior therapists. The behaviorist, therefore, would not view pica as a serious emotional disturbance, but as an unacceptable behavioral habit, specifically as a maladaptive approach response, i.e., an attraction to a behavior that is inappropriate. To clarify, Woody (4) states: "Maladaptive approach responses are those problem behaviors that witness the client's undue attraction to an object, situation, or set of circumstances; these include obsessions and compulsions, homosexuality, alcoholism, and psychological (as opposed to physiological) addiction to drugs. The behavioral modification techniques suitable for maladaptive approach responses, such as pica, include: aversion therapy, clinical suggestion and hypnosis, and covert sensitization.

Aversion Therapy

Aversion therapy or aversive conditioning is a technique that involves the use of unpleasant stimuli to discourage the occurrence of an unacceptable behavior and thus follows a negative reinforcement paradigm. The patient is asked to perform the undesirable act; as he executes it, an unpleasant or aversive stimulus is administered and continues until such a time as the patient stops doing the unacceptable behavioral act. The reward, therefore, occurs when the aversive stimulus stops. In other words, the problem behavior stops, a reward is given (the stopping of the unpleasant stimulus), and the replacing behavioral act, which is acceptable, is perceived as being a welcomed relief from the negative consequences of the target behavioral problem. The technique also involves the concept of punishment since the patient is conditioned to expect punishment when an unacceptable situation arises, and he will be prepared to try to avoid getting into that situation because of the negative expectation.

There are several possible aversive stimuli that are commonly used in behavior therapy, namely, mild electric shock or unpleasant noise or possibly some sort of emetic drug. The first two are usually used with overt behavioral problems, while emetic drugs are usually used with such compulsive acts as alcoholism.

The procedure for using aversive stimuli with a child with pica may be described as follows. The simplest approach would be to present the child with his choice inedible object; as he begins to mouth it, a mild electric shock would be administered. It is feasible that a less distasteful stimulus, such as an unpleasant noise, could be used as well; if this were chosen, it should be administered through ear-phones, in order that the therapist would not also be subjected to the aversive stimulus. After the child had been conditioned to expect the aversive stimulus if he mouthed the object, the shock or noise would be administered whenever he picked up the object and started to bring it toward his mouth. Eventually (and probably after a surprisingly few trials), the child would have a conditioned avoidance response; that is, he would wish to avoid the aversive stimulus and would, therefore, immediately reject the notion to mouth the formerly attractive inedible object.

A slightly more complex procedure would be to involve pictures, such as on 35 mm. slides, of the various acts and objects leading up to the pica behavior. For example, a series of slides could be developed depicting the child (or a model child) looking at the inedible object, touching it, picking it up, fondling it, bringing it toward his mouth, placing it in his mouth, and chewing on it. Pictures of non-pica behaviors would be interspersed between the pica pictures. The child would be allowed to view the pictures (if he were old enough, he would be given control of the automatic changer for switching from one picture to another, such as from a pica picture to a non-pica picture). If he viewed a picture of pica behavior with interest, the aversive stimulus would be administered until he switched the projector to a more acceptable non-pica picture (e.g., of an edible object), at which point the aversive stimulus would stop (in the case of younger children, the therapist would switch the pictures). This procedure would be repeated until the initial pica picture no longer held an attraction for him, a point which could be determined either by asking him (if he were old enough to verbalize) or by recording how quickly he began switching pictures when the target object or pica picture appeared on the screen or by presenting him with the actual inedible object and noting his response (i.e., attracted or repulsed). The second pica picture, which would be designed to allow him even greater identification (psychologically or physically) with the pica behavior, would be shown; then the aversive conditioning process would be repeated until his attraction to this picture was extinguished, and so on.

It should be noted that the aversion therapy can be done with the actual objects, by photographs or pictures, by visual imagery, or by focusing attention on the object via verbal descriptions. In some cases, such as the gnawing on a piece of wood covered by lead paint, it is obvious that it is mandatory that a version other than the actual inedible and harmful object be used. Regardless of presentation mode, the principle is that the negative reactions cultivated by these means will result in a generalization to daily behaviors.

Aversion therapy has proven to be successful in eliminating a wide variety of maladaptive approach responses. Marks (5) and Rachman and Teasdale (6) summarize the research on aversion therapy; further technical descriptions are available in those two sources and elsewhere (4, 7). See Woody (7) for a description of the use of aversion therapy with behavioral problem children.

It is only fair to acknowledge that while aversion therapy does, in fact, appear to be an efficacious treatment approach for maladaptive approach responses, there are many people who would object to its use on the basis of philosophical tenets. In other words, some professionals maintain that aversion therapy has inhumane qualities; behavior therapists, however, assert in return that it is based on a wish to support human integrity, by eliminating a problem behavior that could lead to a chronic handicapping state (or even permanent disability or death as would be the case with lead poisoning). The aversive procedure necessitates that behavior therapists set aside their personal feelings (it is not a pleasant therapeutic procedure for the therapist to administer) in favor of helping patients achieve freedom from the unacceptable problem behaviors. Many behavior therapists openly state that some of their interest in aversive conditioning is rooted in the goal of deriving another treatment approach that is more positive and pleasant (for both the patient and the therapist), but equally as effective as aversion therapy.

Clinical Suggestion and Hypnosis

Clinical suggestion refers to the method in which a professional therapist tries to influence his patient's subsequent behavior by using his professional status to facilitate persuasion relevant to giving up an unacceptable behavior. Clinical suggestion is often incorporated into hypnosis. Woody (4) gives the following definition for hypnosis:

> Hypnosis refers to the state in which the client has achieved a
> degree of relaxation and confidence to allow him to relegate a
> limited command-of-ego-functioning to the counselor-therapist,
> who alters his habituated behaviors, whether attitudinal or acting-

out, by offering suggestions designed to benefit the client and derived from the counselor-therapist's clinical appraisal of the client's functioning and needs.

Induced physical relaxation, through muscular relaxation training, supplements the effects of hypnosis and seems to have a notable value for decreasing intrinsic anxiety by itself; it could, of course, be supplemented by clinical suggestions of decreased anxiety if this were within the therapeutic plan.

Although clinical suggestion and hypnosis are very much a part of many behavior therapy techniques (8), there is reason to question this technique as a sole treatment approach. However, there are numerous published accounts of the success of clinical suggestion and other hypnotic procedures in bringing about marked behavioral changes with at least some children (see for example the *American Journal of Clinical Hypnosis* and the *International Journal of Clinical and Experimental Hypnosis*). But there is reason to wonder whether all children are suitable for such techniques; for example, a major determinant of the success or failure is the relationship between the therapist and the patient (i.e., a strong therapeutic relationship enhances the suggestibility) and with a child with pica it is possible that under usual treatment circumstances, not enough time will have been devoted to building such a relationship; moreover, because of the age of the child it is possible that language communication will also create a barrier.

Covert Sensitization

In the technique of covert sensitization, described initially by Cautela (9), the therapist induces a heightened state of suggestibility, such as through relaxation induction techniques comparable to those used with clinical suggestion and hypnosis; when the patient is in this state, the therapist rigorously helps the patient conjure up an image of himself committing the unacceptable behavioral act and experiencing a disastrous social consequence as a result of it. For example, as the pica child pictures himself eating his favorite inedible object, he would be told to visualize himself being witnessed by his playmates who laugh at and ridicule him; and then as he visualizes himself discarding his inedible object with finality in mind, his playmates are seen as responding positively to him. To date, this technique has had only limited experimentation, but thus far the research data suggest that it has a significant therapeutic potential.

Other Behavioral Techniques

There are several other behavioral techniques that merit mention. These include: negative practice, positive reinforcement via social recognition and object rewards, and behavior shaping.

Negative practice is based on the principle that continued repetition of an undesirable behavioral act will satiate the need for the response's occurrence and it will eventually be extinguished (10, 11). The patient is required to repeat over and over and over the unacceptable behavior with the therapeutic goal being to make the act become totally unrewarding and, in fact, produce a negative effect. Although this technique seems to work with certain problems and with certain types of persons, research on it must be labeled inconclusive. It deserves mention herein because its theoretical properties would be compatible with eliminating pica behavior, but practical matters clearly indicate that it is an unsuitable technique (even if its questionable claim to therapeutic validity and reliability were accepted). Specifically, it seems illogical, to say the least, to require a pica child to ingest vast amounts of inedible, perhaps poisonous, substance!

Positive reinforcement via social recognition and/or object rewards (the latter being either a reward in itself, such as candy, or a token redeemable for prizes or special privileges) has proven to be quite effective for modifying behaviors of both individuals and groups (4, 7). A positive reinforcement paradigm provides for the child's acceptable behavior, such as refusing an inedible object in favor of an edible one, to be rewarded by social recognition (e.g., praise) from a significant person (e.g., the therapist or the child's parents) or a valued object (e.g., tokens that could be accumulated and redeemed for a toy). But if the child demonstrates an unacceptable behavior, such as giving preference to an inedible object, the same reinforcements—social recognition and object rewards—are withheld or withdrawn. Withdrawing a previously given reward takes on a punishing quality. While this technique has theoretical suitability for pica and would in all likelihood promote change toward giving priority to edible objects rather than inedible ones it has the drawback of producing relatively slower results, as compared to aversion therapy, clinical suggestion and hypnosis and covert sensitization; and with a pica child it is critical that a prompt change be accomplished, as it could be disastrous for him to keep ingesting the inedible materials. It seems, however, that positive reinforcement via social recognition and object rewards have a definite place in the behavioral modification of the pica child. Specifically, these positive reinforcements, while being used in the actual therapy sessions, could also be implemented at home by the child's parents. By training the parents to participate in the behavioral modification program, it is possible to eliminate any subtle (or not so subtle) inappropriate reinforcers that the parents might be sending out that would actually encourage the child's pica behavior; for example, and in accord with one of the possible etiologies of pica, some children become starved for affect from their parents and the only way they get any affect is to arouse negative affect by engaging in a behavior (such as pica) that upsets their parents.

Behavior shaping has been described in detail by Bandura and Walters (12). In this technique, the child views certain key behaviors (in films or actuality) that are structured so as to lead him to alter his own unacceptable behavior. Usually, the principle of successive approximation is employed. For example, the patient might view filmed episodes depicting a child similar to himself engaged in a behavior just about like that of the patient (but slightly more acceptable), with successive episodes depicting behaviors that are progressively more acceptable. The child in the film might also be shown receiving reinforcements, such as social recognition and/or object rewards. Thus the patient presumably identifying with the film model, would be prone to behave in the manner shown in the films, initially aiming at the behavior that was just about like his but slightly better; and in each of the trials, he would harbor the expectation that he will be rewarded, as was the model, when he behaves in a like manner. In some instances, the film model may be shown receiving punishment for an unacceptable behavior, and this kind of scene would, of course, lead the patient-viewer to anticipate the same sort of negative consequences if he behaved in the same unacceptable way.

Although films (or video tape recordings) are commonly used in clinical settings, it is also feasible, and perhaps more practical, to involve actual children; in other words, one or more peers might be engaged in performing certain key behaviors in the presence of the patient, with care being taken to have a progressive sequence of models (moving from behaviors quite similar to the present status of the patient to behaviors that progressively improve). As was the case with positive reinforcement via social recognition and object rewards behavior shaping has theoretical compatibility with pica behavior but also has the characteristic of proceeding more slowly and being more reliant upon facilities and resources (it is admittedly difficult to arrange for appropriate films and/or children to produce the modeling behavior) than for aversion therapy, clinical suggestion and hypnosis, and covert sensitization. Again, however, this may be a suitable adjunctive technique, e.g., having children spurn inedible materials for modeling effects.

DISCUSSION

The foregoing discussion touches on two topics that deserve elaboration. First it seems advisable to reinspect the existing two theories of the etiology of pica and to attempt to establish an explanation for the development of pica according to learning theory. Second, attention should be given to reconciling theoretical positions and bridging the gap from the present "renovation" posture to the more desirable "environmental-psychobehavioral" posture.

TOWARD A BEHAVIORAL ETIOLOGICAL CONCEPTUALIZATION OF PICA

As mentioned previously, the two basic etiological explanations of pica posit a nutritional deficit and a psychosexual developmental conflict. The first assumes that the behavior is a consequence of a nutritional deficit and that that child is trying to compensate by actively ingesting, almost indiscriminately perhaps, inedible substances. The second, which is primarily psychodynamic, posits that the child-mother relationship has not been adequate enough to fulfill the child's need for affection and that the resulting insecurity leads him to the inept mode of compensation called pica. These two theories receive wide acceptance, though neither has been thoroughly researched and neither has more than speculative validation. Both theories are directed mainly at the young child (younger than five years of age), and treatment recommendations are rather superficial. For example, note the following total recommendation excerpted from one contemporary text on behavioral problem children; Verville (1) states:

> More nutritious food should be given the child with pica, and inedible substances should be cleaned up or kept out of his reach. He must be closely supervised so that he can be restrained from consuming forbidden matter and offered food instead. Playing with the child each day provides him with the personal attention he often has lacked. (p. 139)

As will be evident in the ensuing discussion, this kind of recommendation is much too superficial to counteract adequately the forces operating within the pica child, and certain elements of the recommendation (such as giving "close supervision" and giving a "forbidden" connotation to his behavior) could actually serve to reinforce the pica behavior.

Pica in older children (e.g., elementary school children in the age range of 5 to 12 years) also occurs. In these instances, the tendency seems to be to give priority to the psychodynamic etiological explanation; Verville (1) states:

> This behavior is not comparable to the pica of the pre-school child, who experiments from curiosity or undernourishment. Older children punish themselves in this way or use themselves as substitutes for parents they believe to be deserving of punishment.
> . . . Deliberate and drastic self-harm warns parents of serious disturbance in the child. The child needs increased physical affection and attention, and anger directed against him and against the other parent should be curtailed. As the family tension decreases and the child is able to regain some trust in his parents, he should be encouraged to talk about his worries and ask questions, even though

these are embarrassing or accusatory. The parents need to settle their differences and provide assurance to the child that the family is not disintegrating. (p. 222)

Again it is evident that the treatment intervention proposed is rather superficial, although the connotation is clearly that insight oriented counseling and psychotherapy is necessary for the child and his family in total. From a psychodynamic viewpoint, it is regrettable that the environmental manipulation includes a curtailing of the expression of key emotions, such as anger; the expression of these emotions is tantamount to eventually gaining resolution for the underlying emotional conflicts and for developing improved coping behaviors. Parenthetically, it is important to note that the last two treatment proposals were selected as being representative of the current professional thinking, and they should not be lightly passed over as derived from an inferior reference source (the source seems, in fact, superior to many of its counterparts).

To summarize the theoretical aspects discussed to this point, both etiological explanations of pica are commonly interpreted as supporting the need for a prompt altering of the physical environment, such as by renovating the house in which the child with lead poisoning lives, and urging somewhat coercive or directive guidance from the adults within the child's life space. This is the situation for children regardless of age or point of onset of the pica behavior. There is only a secondary emphasis on actually trying to deal with the possibility of psychodynamic conflicts.

A behavioral conceptualization of the etiology of pica, regardless of the age of the child, is much more simple: it would appear that pica behavior is learned. In other words, whether for nutritional or psychodynamic reasons (or perhaps even by chance occurrence alone), the child ingests an inedible object (or substance) and finds that it brings some reward, perhaps a reduction in his anxiety about his relationship with his mother or his insecurity or a physiological craving, and because he found it satisfying (i.e., reinforcing), he tends to repeat the behavior again. Such behavior might be repeated even though the original reason for its occurrence had long since disappeared or had been dissipated (perhaps the mother had subsequently given the child more affection); the child might associate the initial pica act with his subsequent increased maternal affective reward or he might just recall that it had given him pleasure at one time—and so it is perpetuated.

A ready analogy can be found with the development of fetishes—and in a manner of speaking, pica assumes the characteristics of a fetish: the person with a fetish, upon introspecting about its evolution during psychotherapy, usually comes up with a remembrance of how his first few trials of using his favored object in conjunction with emotional, often sexual, gratification were accompanied by a significant decrease in anxiety, insecurity or emotional and/or physical discomfort, and later in life, such as when he is an adult with other presumably more satisfying outlets (e.g., being heterosexual and having good sexual relations with his wife), the person still finds his fetish rewarding. Admittedly, persons with fetishes, and probably some children with pica can often identify how the initial inappropriate object-behavioral choice came to be selected almost by chance, but was done in a moment of emotional crisis.

The acquisition of pica behavior is in many ways comparable to the acquisition of fetish behavior (whether overtly sexualized or not): the inappropriate chosen objects or substances provide emotional gratification. In other words, there is a reward which leads to the behavior being reinforced. Further, it is quite possible that the inappropriate behavior, while having reinforcement value when initially relied upon, can also provoke reactions from others that will give additional reinforcement. As was mentioned earlier, the child who eats an inedible object or substance, and such an act may or may not be rewarding in and of itself, often discovers that the act alarms significant others (e.g., his parents) and suddenly he receives all kinds of attention and affect—which, though perhaps negative (e.g., anger), is still the much coveted affect—from professionals (who scamper around because of the possible emergency) and from his parents, and such reactions, especially from his parents, may be of particular importance to a child. Thus a child who senses a lack of affect in his relationship with his parents might find the affective exclamations and actions of his parents in regard to his pica behavior to be reinforcing and he would consequently be prone to repeat it.

Professionals with a psychoanalytic orientation might also want to point to the reinforcement of an undesired effect, albeit symbolic, associated with the typical environmental renovation plan. For the child who has a conflict about his feelings for his parents, such as the boy with Oedipal feelings for his mother or the girl with Electra feelings for her father, both of whom have guilt feelings (usually subconscious) and fear of the opposite parent, there is great symbolic value in the ingestion of the physical environment and the resulting renovating actions of others. Fenichel (13) states: "If oral impulses have been subjected to specific repressions, a frequent result is in an inhibition of eating, or of eating certain kinds of food which are unconsciously reminiscent of the objects desired by the repressed oral-erotic strivings" (p. 175). From a psychoanalytic point of view, what would have more symbolic import than the ingestion of the environment that is unsatisfying, that is frustrating and cannot be effectively controlled, and that produces conflicting feelings. The implication is: "look how powerful I am, I can gradually eliminate everything by eating it." And to the psychoanalyst, of course, eating or oral gratification has a direct relationship with psychosexual or erotic gratification. Further, there is psychoanalytic significance in the environmental renovations. Again what could have more psychic import than to have other persons, such as doctors who are more powerful than the feared (yet loved) parents, press the parents into a cooperative effort to tear the physical environment apart and rebuild it—perhaps not to the specifications of the pica child but at least because of him. The important thing within this psychoanalytic interpretation is that there are reinforcers being accorded to the child because of his unacceptable pica behavior. While the danger of a particular substance can be eliminated, such as removal of lead-based paint, at the same time there is a presetting of the child for using other unacceptable behaviors, and perhaps even the pica, at some point in the future. For optimal success over the child's life time, the circumstances surrounding the pica behavior must be deprived of reinforcements toward unacceptable behavior and efforts taken to help the child to deal more effectively with the emotional factors that might have prompted it in the first place.

TOWARD AN ENVIRONMENTAL-PSYCHOBEHAVIORAL POSTURE

As repeatedly stated, the current most prominent approach to intervening to eliminate pica behavior is environmental alteration. For example, in cases in which children develop lead poisoning from pica behavior associated with ingesting lead-based paint particles, their homes, which are typically older dilapidated houses, are thoroughly scraped down, with perhaps whole walls being replaced, and repainted. Not only is the cost restrictive, it may even be unnecessary for the most part, and there are theoretical reasons for questioning whether this form of environmental change accomplishes anything related to the etiology of the pica behavior. In the cases where, following the renovation of the house, the child does not repeat the pica behavior, both behaviorally and psychoanalytically oriented professionals would concur that this "cure" could be due to the child's finding a more satisfactory way to fulfill his needs, that the precipitating need may have lost its prominence in the child's behavioral repertoire by virtue of having already served its purpose and a different (new) but psychodynamically related unacceptable behavioral manifestation may be occurring instead, or that significant others might be giving him undeserved reinforcers, such as either positive or negative affect, because of the *coup d'état* that his pica behavior created.

Regarding the theories of the pica behavior, it is clearly evident that whether one primarily accepts the nutritional, psychodynamic, or behavioral conceptualization (and it is, of course, feasible that more than one, if not all, has validity, depending upon the child and the circumstances), there is little to support that an intervention involving solely an environmental alteration has truly curative properties. What is needed is an augmentation for the environmental approach, namely methods that will attempt to resolve the inferred emotional conflicts and that will control inept reinforcers. This would, of course, be in addition to a comprehensive medical evaluation designed to ascertain the possible influence of a real nutritional deficit or some organic dysfunctioning.

In view of the pronounced possibility that each of the etiological conceptualizations has application to at least a portion of children with pica, it is essential to define the therapeutic intervention in such a manner as to accommodate quite diverse psychodynamic and behavioristic tenets. Despite the fact that the insight oriented approaches to counseling and psychotherapy decry the behavioristic notion that problems are maladaptive learned responses and that the behaviorists in turn dispute the assumption of an underlying emotional conflict for behavioral problems, there is evidence that supports, much like the comments on the validity of the different etiological conceptualizations for pica, that certain behavioral problems are rooted in psychodynamic conflicts, others in purely faulty or maladaptive learning, and others in a combination (4, 7, 14, 15). Logically, the most versatile and comprehensive therapeutic intervention would, therefore, embrace both the insight oriented (i.e., psychodynamically based) techniques of counseling and psychotherapy and the behaviorally oriented (i.e., conditioning based) techniques of behavior therapy. Indeed, despite seeming contradictions, there is clinical and experimental evidence to support that insight and behavioral approaches have both theoretical and technical compatibility (4, 7, 14, 15, 16). Woody (4, 7, 14) has labeled this integrative approach the *Psychobehavioral* frame of reference. Admittedly, behavioral techniques have been heretofore by-passed in the treatment of pica behavior, but theoretical compatibility and clinical-experimental research with related behavioral disorders provide strong support for their potential value.

Bridging the gap from the present "renovation" posture to the more desirable and hopefully more efficacious "environmental-psychobehavioral" posture is not actually an unreasonable task, neither in terms of theory nor practicality. It can be reduced to the postulate: *the condition of pica can best be treated by the combined services of medical and mental health personnel.* This underscores the importance of the physical-mental-environmental forces that act upon a child, and supports that the professional personnel involved with the child displaying pica behavior should be able to offer preventive recommendations, environmental alterations, medical diagnostics and treatments, and psychobehavioral counseling and therapy accordingly. It is only through such an interdisciplinary stance that the necessary theoretical and technical eclecticism can be accommodated.

SUMMARY

Existing theories of pica, namely that pica is due to a nutritional deficit or a psychosexual emotional conflict, have not been validated, and there is reason to believe that a third etiological theory, aligned with behaviorism, might be equally justifiable. Treatment of the pica child and especially children who have ingested significant amounts of lead-based materials have been relatively ineffective. Moreover, certain elements of the crisis oriented approach to the treatment, from the exaggerated affect of both parents and professionals to the physical rennovation of the child's home environment (supposedly to eliminate the possibility of further lead poisoning), could serve to reinforce the pica behavior (particularly if the hypothesized psychosexual elements are present) and thus might actually be deleterious actions. It would appear that behavioral modification techniques have been too long bypassed in the treatment of pica, and that the most appropriate treatment would be an integrated environmental-psychobehavioral approach.

REFERENCES

1. Verville, Elinor. *Behavior Problems of Children*. Philadelphia: W. B. Saunders, 1967.
2. Kanner, L. *Child Psychiatry* (3rd ed.). Springfield, Ill.: C. C. Thomas, 1957.
3. Kessler, Jane W. *Psychopathology of Childhood*. Englewood Cliffs, N.J.: Prentice-Hall, 1966.
4. Woody, R. H. *Psychobehavioral Counseling and Therapy Integrating Behavioral and Insight Techniques*. New York: Appleton-Century-Crofts, 1971.
5. Marks, I. M. Aversion therapy. *British Journal of Medical Psychology*, 1968, *41*, 47-52.
6. Rachman, S., and Teasdale, J. *Aversion Therapy and Behavior Disorders: An Analysis*. Coral Gables, Fla.: University of Miami Press, 1969.
7. Woody, R. H. *Behavioral Problem Children in the Schools: Recognition, Diagnosis, and Behavioral Modification*. New York: Appleton-Century-Crofts, 1969.
8. Klein, Marjorie H., Dittmann, A. T., Parloff, M. B., and Gill, M. M. Behavior therapy: Observations and reflections. *Journal of Consulting and Clinical Psychology*, 1969, *33*, 259-266.
9. Cautela, J. R. Covert sensitization. *Psychological Report*, 1967, *20*, 459-468.
10. Dunlap, K. *Habits, Their Making and Unmaking*. New York: Liveright, 1932.
11. Lehner, G. F. J. Negative practice as a psychotherapeutic technique. In H. J. Eysenck (ed.), *Behaviour Therapy and the Neuroses*. New York: Pergamon, 1960, pp. 194-206.
12. Bandura, A., and Walters, R. H. *Social Learning and Personality Development*. New York: Holt, Rinehart and Winston, 1963.
13. Fenichel, O. *The Psychoanalytic Theory of Neurosis*. New York: W. W. Norton, 1945.

14. Woody, R. H. Toward a rationale for psychobehavioral therapy. *Archives of General Psychiatry*, 1968, *19*, 197-204.
15. Marks, I. M., and Gelder, M. G. Common ground between behavior therapy and psychodynamic methods. *British Journal of Medical Psychology*, 1966, *39*, 11-23.
16. Mowrer, O. H. Freudianism, behaviour therapy and "self-disclosure." *Behaviour Research and Therapy*, 1964, *1*, 321-337.

12

WEIGHT

INTRODUCTION

Obesity

Childhood obesity can be defined as an excess amount of body fat that has an adverse effect on the social functioning of the child or on current and future health (Weil, 1977). At least 17 percent of males and 12 percent of females are obese by age 13 (USDHEW, 1972). The incidence rate is higher among lower socioeconomic status groups (Stunkard, 1977). Since over 80 percent of overweight children become overweight adults (Abraham & Nordsieck, 1960), effective treatment or prevention during childhood may be critical.

Only a small percentage of childhood obesity is now attributed solely to physiological disorders; the role of metabolic and genetic differences and the factors that control eating and activity behaviors are being explored (Mayer, 1975). How these possible causes interact is still largely unknown. For example, less eating or more exercise will definitely lead to fat loss, but physiological factors may make dieting or activity highly aversive and thus not maintained over a sufficiently long period to have a significant effect (Foreyt, Goodrick, & Gotto, 1981). Approaches used traditionally have been notoriously ineffective: diets, anorectic drugs, traditional exercise programs, therapeutic starvation, and even bypass surgery have been shown to be ineffective in producing lasting weight loss in children, to say nothing of the possible dangers and side effects of such treatments (Coates & Thoresen, 1978).

There have been only a few behavioral attempts to produce weight loss in obese children. Aragona, Cassady, and Drabman (1975) trained parents in the use of exercise, nutrition, stimulus control of eating, and reinforcement for appropriate behaviors with their overweight children. Parents whose children failed to meet weight goals forfeited deposit money. Kingsley and Shapiro (1977) had parents use stimulus control, self-monitoring, and a token-economy system to modify their children's eating and exercise behaviors. Dinoff, Rickard, and Colwick (1972) obtained a good weight loss in an obese boy by using a contractual agreement between the boy and a camp counselor, which stipulated reduced food intake and rewards for compliance. These studies have shown weight loss in the short term. However, recent reviews (Brownell & Stunkard, 1978; Coates & Thoresen, 1978) have pointed out that losses are usually not maintained one year later. Thus the results of behavioral treatment of obesity in children parallel those for adults: behavioral methods produce the best short-term losses, but the weight returns (Stunkard & Penick, 1979). There is mounting evidence that a focus on behavioral treatment of obesity for children should be exercise programs integrated into the school system, using carefully graduated aerobic exercise (Foreyt & Goodrick, in press). If properly presented, such programs could be enjoyed by most children and may lead to long-term weight regulation as well as a higher level of physical fitness.

The study by Wheeler and Hess (1976) in this chapter focuses mainly on eating behavior, but includes lack of exercise as a problem area. The successive approximation technique used demonstrates how a parent can identify problems such as overeating or hypoactivity, and then use stimulus control, substitution, and reinforcement to change the child's behaviors. Perhaps if such a treatment were expanded to include monitoring of food and increased exercise in the school setting, results would be more impressive and longer lasting.

Anorexia Nervosa

Anorexia nervosa is insufficient eating behavior resulting in unhealthful weight loss. It is characterized by a reported loss of appetite in the absence of organic causes or psychosis. Most cases begin in early adolescence, with the syndrome more common among females. The incidence among adolescent girls may be as high as four per 1,000 (Crisp, 1979).

In some cases voluntary vomiting may occur to further reduce nutritional uptake (Scrignar, 1971). Since the health hazards can be severe, hospitalization and medical interventions such as tube feeding and drug therapy are often used immediately. However, the effects of traditional treatment in the hospital may not generalize to the home situation (Liebman, Minuchin & Baker, 1974) and no effective medical treatments have been recognized (Halmi, 1978).

The behavioral approach used most often is reinforcement for eating and weight gain. A review by Bhanji and Thompson (1974) cites a number of studies in which hospitalized patients were allowed privileges such as parental visits, television, or out-of-room activity contingent upon weight gain. Werry and Bull (1975) extended such contingencies to the home; lack of weight improvement meant a return to the hospital. Agras, Barlow, Chapin, Abel, and Leitenberg (1974), in a series of single case experiments, found that effective variables for treatment include negative reinforcement through removal from bleak hospital surroundings contingent upon weight gain, positive reinforcement with desired activities, and information feedback about calories consumed and weight gain so that the adolescent can learn when to expect reinforcement; making it more effective. They also found that larger meals resulted in more being eaten.

Behavioral studies performed only in the hospital setting have shown disappointing long-term results (Siegel & Richards, 1978). Bruch (1974) has criticized several behavioral studies that showed rapid weight loss when treatment ended. She feels that this is due to the failure both to treat the underlying psychological problems and to follow the patients after treatment. In the study in this chapter, a combination of family therapy and behavioral techniques were used for a more complete treatment. The approach used by Liebman, Minuchin, and Baker (1974) begins with contingency management in the hospital and ends with family therapy in the home. The four girls treated had to gain weight each week in order to visit friends or have friends over on the weekend. This study illustrates how a pediatrician and a psychiatrist coordinated the treatment program in the hospital and home, respectively. The emphasis on family contingencies allowed maintenance of appropriate behaviors and attainment of normal weight in the home setting.

References

Abraham, S., & Nordsieck, M. Relationship of excess weight in children and adults. *Public Health Reports*, 1960, *75*, 263-273.

Agras, W. S., Barlow, D. H., Chapin, H. N., Abel, G. G., & Leitenberg, H. Behavior modification of anorexia nervosa. *Archives of General Psychiatry*, 1974, *30*, 279-286.

Aragona, J., Cassady, J., & Drabman, R. S. Treating overweight children through parental training and contingency contracting. *Journal of Applied Behavior Analysis*, 1975, *8*, 269-278.

Bhanji, S., & Thompson, J. Operant conditioning in the treatment of anorexia nervosa: A review and retrospective study of 11 cases. *British Journal of Psychiatry*, 1974, *124*, 166-172

Brownell, K. D., & Stunkard, A. J. Behavioral treatment of obesity in children. *American Journal of Diseases of Children*, 1978, *132*, 403-412.

Bruch, H. Perils of behavior modification in treatment of anorexia nervosa. *Journal of The American Medical Association*, 1974, *230*, 1419-1422.

Coates, T. J., & Thoresen, C. E. Treating obesity in children and adolescents: A review. *American Journal of Public Health*. 1978, *68*, 143-151.

Crisp, A. H. Early recognition and prevention of anorexia nervosa. *Developmental Medicine and Child Neurology*, 1979, *21*, 393-395.

Dinoff, M., Rickard, H. C., & Colwick, J. Weight reduction through successive contracts. *American Journal of Orthopsychiatry*, 1972, *42*, 110-113.

Foreyt, J. P., & Goodrick, G. K. Assessment of childhood obesity. In E. Mash & L. Terdal (Eds.), *Behavior assessment of childhood disorders.* New York: Guilford Press, in press.

Foreyt, J. P., Goodrick, G. K., & Gotto, A. M. Behavioral treatment of obesity. *Journal of Behavioral Medicine*, 1981, *4*, in press.

Halmi, K. A. Anorexia nervosa: Recent investigations. *Annual Review of Medicine*, 1978, *29*, 137-148.

Kingsley, R. G., & Shapiro, J. A comparison of three behavioral programs for the control of obesity in children. *Behavior Therapy*, 1977, *8*, 30-36.

Liebman, R., Minuchin, S., & Baker, L. An integrated treatment program for anorexia nervosa. *American Journal of Psychiatry*, 1974, *131*, 432-436.

Mayer, J. Obesity during childhood. In M. Winick (Ed.), *Childhood obesity.* New York: John Wiley & Sons, 1975.

Scrignar, C. B. Food as the reinforcer in the outpatient treatment of anorexia nervosa. *Journal of Behavior Therapy and Experimental Psychiatry*, 1971, *2*, 31-36.

Siegel, L. J., & Richards, C. S. Behavioral intervention with somatic disorders in children. In D. Marholin II (Ed.), *Child Behavior Therapy.* New York: Gardner Press, Inc., 1978, 339-394.

Stunkard, A. J. Obesity and the social environment: Current status, future prospects. *Annals of the New York Academy of Science*, 1977, *300*, 298-320.

Stunkard, A. J., & Penick, S. B. Behavior modification in the treatment of obesity: The problem of maintaining weight loss. *Archives of General Psychiatry*, 1979, *36*, 801-806.

U.S. Department of Health, Education, and Welfare. *Ten state nutrition survey.* Department of Health, Education, and Welfare Publication No. (HSM) 73-8704. Washington, D.C.: U.S. Government Printing Office, 1972.

Weil, W. B. Current controversies in childhood obesity. *Journal of Pediatrics*, 1977, *91*, 175-187.

Werry, J. S., & Bull, D. Anorexia nervosa: A case study using behavior therapy. *Journal of the American Academy of Child Psychiatry*, 1975, *14*, 646-651.

Wheeler, M. E., & Hess, K. W. Treatment of juvenile obesity by successive approximation control of eating. *Journal of Behavior Therapy and Experimental Psychiatry*, 1976, 7, 235-241.

TREATMENT OF JUVENILE OBESITY
BY SUCCESSIVE APPROXIMATION
CONTROL OF EATING

Mary Ebel Wheeler
Karl W. Hess

Summary—A group of mother-child pairs received behavioral treatment for juvenile obesity. The treatment children, aged 2-10,
outperformed untreated controls, and striking differences in movement toward appropriate weight-for-age-and height norms were
found between those remaining in the program and those who
dropped out. The program involved a long term successive
approximation approach to control of eating patterns within the
family and social context of the patient. Emphasis was placed
upon the individualization of treatment.

A variety of evidence points to the need for treatment programs designed
specifically for obese juveniles (Knittle, 1971; Wolff, 1955; Mayer, 1968).
Not only are the psychological roots of much of adult obesity to be found in
childhood, but there are data that suggest that cellular composition in early
onset obesity is different from that arising in later obesities. This may provide
a physiological block to effective treatment, which, added to the evidence that
food preferences and habits are developed early in life, argues for effective
treatment of obesity in the child.

Reprinted from *Journal of Behavior Therapy and Experimental Psychiatry*, 1976,
7, 235-241. Copyright 1976 by Pergamon Press Ltd. Reprinted by permission.

Mary Ebel Wheeler is presently at the Center for Optimal Growth of Kaiser-
Permanente in Cleveland Heights, Ohio. Karl W. Hess is in the Psychology Department
of Case Western Reserve in Cleveland, Ohio.

This investigation was supported in full by the U.S. Public Health Service Biomedical Research Support Grant #2 507 RR5221 to Kaiser Foundation Research Institute
and the Kaiser Foundation Hospitals.

Programs reported by previous investigators have generally been of two types: (1) dietary with or without amphetamine supplementation (Asher, 1966; Lloyd et al., 1961), or (2) combinations of diet and exercise (Rohrbacher, 1973; Parizkova et al., 1962; Pekos, 1960). These latter programs are most often conducted at summer camps, although some have been implemented in schools (Christakis et al., 1966). The results of these studies are impossible to compare. The degree and duration of initial obesity varies vastly among programs, and even indicators such as dropout rates are difficult to compare because of diverse treatment durations and differences in patient selection and motivation. Previous investigations, especially those conducted in clinical settings, generally have dealt with children who are (1) grossly obese, typically above the 95th percentile for their height and age, (2) have obesity of long standing, and (3) are adolescent or older. The present study applied a behavioral treatment program to a sample of less obese, younger children in an attempt to determine if this was a possible avenue of control for juvenile obesity, as it has been with adults (Stuart and Davis, 1972).

It should be noted that there are striking differences between obesity programs for adults and for children. In children, especially those below the ages of five, a change in the child (e.g., weight loss and more appropriate eating) may be effected primarily through modification of maternal behaviors. Such programs necessitate a family-oriented approach. The present pilot program carried out through the Kaiser Health Foundation facility in Cleveland, Ohio, built upon this recognition with the avowed intention of arriving at a re-education of eating habits through a combination of parent-child management.

Behavioral control of childhood obesity has several points of difference in relation to traditional dietary approaches including:

1. Emphasis upon the analysis of the stimuli surrounding and maintaining excess eating, rather than upon simple curtailment of calories.

2. Identification and manipulation of the rewards which support over-eating, including those which stem from social and familial circumstances.

3. Involvement of the child and parent as active participants in the process of arriving at a more suitable eating pattern.

4. Recognition of the necessity for gradual approximation to a goal, with emphasis upon movement toward that goal rather than upon reaching a preset dietary prescription.

The essential element of this approach is the dynamic relation between analysis and change—leading to an individualization of treatment and the possibility of permanent change through re-education.

ASSESSMENT

Analysis of the stimuli in and around the eating situation was crucial to diagnosing possible foci for change. The principal tool employed was the Food Intake Record, a patient report form concerned with the identification of where food was eaten, the social surroundings in which it was eaten, the time of its ingestion, and the amount eaten, as well as the specific foods involved. This record calls attention to patterns of behavior that may not have been previously noted by the parent. It also provides information pertinent to the identification of possible points of control. Children who make their own breakfast and dinner require different controls than those who are served these meals by a parent.

ALTERATION

Table 12.1 describes eight of the most common problems encountered in this project and some of the alternative controls employed. Which of these solutions was employed depended upon its physical feasibility in the child's environment, as well as the parent's reaction to it. The problems focused on were limited to one or two at each treatment session. A subjective judgment was made of problems that seemed most aggravating and most amenable to change. Some problems could not be effectively dealt with in a specific family context (e.g., eating high caloric ethnic foods).

ADJUSTMENT

Changes were evaluated at the session subsequent to their implementation. The efficacy of a procedure was determined from weight loss, the Food Intake Record, and patient report. Since the key to the success of our procedures rested in large measure with the parents, emphasis was placed upon discussion of their views of the course of treatment. In many cases it may be that the key difference between our approach and that of others was the motivational consequence of our repeated contact with the mother. Changes in treatment were introduced when weight loss was not apparent or patient dissatisfaction was reported. No attempt was made to persist in procedures that proved uncomfortable as the probability of these leading to long-term change seemed low. The focus was upon a constantly evolving situation that was practical for the given patient in his particular environment.

TABLE 12.1. Changes in eating made during treatment

| Problem behaviors | Situations | | | Consequences |
	Eliminate inappropriate	Control inappropriate	Provide appropriate	Provide positive
1. Child consumes large amounts of candy, cookies, and ice cream	Eliminate such foods from home	But food in portion controlled sizes for clear record of amount	Less caloric but attractive snacks	Select one food as daily treat for appropriate eating
		Use outside source (ice cream truck, walk to store) for treats		
2. Child eats "on the run"—snacking from kitchen	Kitchen off bounds	Set times for snack same time every day	Bin of snacks easily accessible and of low calorie	Occasional favored snack placed in bin
	Tempting foods locked away or eliminated	Child given "out of house" activities during difficult times	Substitute lower calorie snacks	
3. Child eats overly large quantities of food at meals	Mother dishes up plates in kitchen	Mother provides seconds of vegetables and salads first	Meal begins with child's less favored food (salad first)	Child gets money or token for leaving food on plate
4. Child must prepare own food (changes difficult)	Child's responsibilities change	Mother prepares frozen dinners or buys low calorie ones	Child cooks low calorie foods	
		Child cooks with sibling		

Problem				
5. Child consuming food for which less caloric substitutes are available	End purchases of high caloric foods	Buy lower calorie foods	Educate concerning the problems or possibilities of alternate foods	Reward mother for following suggestions and devising her own
6. Child gets no exercise	Curtail TV and other sedentary activities	Schedule TV viewing	Develop new exercise child enjoys	Make treat contingent upon certain "countable" activities
			Revise family activities	Involve parent in shared activity
7. Parents are "fair" and share with child their inappropriate eating	Eliminate inappropriate food from child's world	Parents' inappropriate eating changed to outside home	Parent cooks special treat for special child	Reinforce "different treatment"
			Incorporate low risk foods into family diet	
8. High incidence of party or outside home eating (baby-sitter)	Restrict parties	Have mother inform others about child'd difficulty or have office visit	Select and save for treat at home one special food	
		Request limitations of availability of inappropriate food		

Note: The problems listed are the eight most frequent problems listed in all records, both treatment and dropout.

Success in this sort of treatment is tied closely to careful analysis and record keeping. The individualization of treatment hinges upon the therapist's ability to keep track of, and reliably recall, the circumstances of a patient's life. Since our program involved analysis of the home setting and the specific stimuli for eating, it is apparent that a microanalysis of the patient's eating behaviors was called for. The Food Intake Record was designed to implement this analysis and was augmented by detailed notes made during each session. Specifically, the program involved:

1. Detailed analysis of the stimuli and rewards associated with eating in the child's home environment, through the use of the Food Intake Record during a 2-week pretreatment baseline measurement. The patient or parent indicated all eating activity during the pretreatment period and for at least the first several weeks of treatment.

2. Specific and limited manipulations of components of eating judged to be especially disruptive or counterproductive, with limited specific manipulations, e.g. limitation of TV snacking, in any one treatment session.

3. Follow-up of the effect of each manipulation through weight change and patient report at each subsequent session, with considerable emphasis upon the maintenance of parent interest and commitment. In particular, any slowing of weight gain received praise and reiteration of the importance of early control of what could be a life-long problem.

4. Gradual accretion of controls until a stable and satisfactory system suited to long-term control of the child's intake could be achieved. This approximation was realized by the reaching of a state where there was constant movement toward a satisfactory weight, and in which there was a controlled intake mechanism.

5. Assumption of the responsibility for analysis and control by the mother and child, in the hope of effecting real re-education.

METHODS

Subjects

Forty children between the ages of 2 and 11 were obtained by referral from the population at the Kaiser Permanente Facility on the east side of Cleveland, Ohio. Pediatricians were invited to refer patients of obvious obesity but without medical or psychological disorder. The program was offered without charge to medical plan subscribers.

Subject skinfold thicknesses ranged from one to nine standard deviations above the mean for their age, sex, and race (median = 3.0 standard deviations). An attempt was made to admit children from a reasonably broad age range and degree of obesity (mean age at program onset = 7.1 yr).

Procedure

The population of suitable subjects was divided into experimental and control groups as they were referred for treatment. The assignment was random, with the limitation that preference was given to the treatment condition for the first child referred in each category under study. The control group was never contacted.

The final distribution of patients is presented in Table 12.2. Of the 40 subjects, those 12 patients who dropped out of treatment after three or fewer treatment sessions were considered dropouts. Fourteen remained in treatment for 4 or more sessions and constitute the *treatment* condition, while an additional 14 patients who were never contacted made up the *control* group.

The apparently higher percentage of females in the treatment group reflects the lower number of females who dropped the program. Since Kaiser records do not contain information on race, it was impossible to determine the racial character of the control group.

During the initial contact, previously developed instruments recording family situation and food preferences were completed by the mother. The child's weight, height, skinfold thicknesses, and three semi-nude pictures (dorsal, ventral, and lateral) were obtained, as well as recordings of blood pressure and serum cholesterol level. The Food Intake Record was explained and given to the parent (and child) to complete during the next two weeks. At each subsequent visit, height and weight were obtained, and skinfold thickness were measured periodically during treatment.

Treatment involved mother-child pairs in individual half-hour sessions. Initially the sessions were at two-week intervals, but were gradually spaced

TABLE 12.2. Comparison of group age, sex, race, and percent overweight

	Treatment (n = 14)	Drop-out (n = 12)	Control (n = 14)
Mean average years	7.6	6.3	7.4
Female %(n)	79% (9)	42% (5)	50% (7)
Black %(n)	64% (9)	83% (10)	—
Mean percent overweight			
At onset	40.4	46.3	38.9
Last data point	34.9	52.1	44.4
Change*	−4.1	+3.0	+6.3

*Mean individual change for matched treatment and controls and available dropouts.

further apart if progress was being made. Parents were encouraged to become independent and make appointments according to their needs. Thus, after progress had begun and was proceeding well, visits were often at 3-week or longer intervals.

RESULTS

Treatment Success

In dealing with a growing organism, the specification of a criterion of weight adjustment is difficult. While pounds-lost is the traditional adult measure, it can be deceptive even with the relatively stable patterns of adulthood (Mayer, 1968). Since this program sought to deal with the rapidly growing child, pounds-lost would only poorly reflect the child's actual relation to mean weight for height, age, and sex, since these norms would change over the course of treatment. Thus, change in percentage overweight was selected as the most sensitive measure available to assess change in obesity. Differences between a child's actual weight and the mean weight for his height, sex and age (USD-HEW Vital and Health Statistics) were computed before and after a uniform period of treatment (or nontreatment in the control condition). These differences were expressed as percentage overweights.

While the percentage overweight might possibly reflect an excess of muscle as well as fatty tissue (Mayer, 1968), it should be noted that skinfold thickness also served as criteria for inclusion in the program—therefore substantiating the obese composition of the sample. Success, for the purposes of this study, was defined as being closer to mean weight for age, sex, and height at the end of the study period than at the beginning. Since patients were added to the sample as they were referred or as others dropped out, some of the treatment durations were brief and the percentage changes relatively modest. Calculation of percentage overweight for the dropout and control patients was made at the time of the last medical visit—whether for our study or for any other medical reason.

Of the 26 patients contacted initially, 12 (46%) dropped out after four or fewer sessions. Of the remaining children, 10 (71%) were closer to their appropriate weight at the completion of the study than at the onset and four (28%) were further away from their appropriate weights. Overall comparison of the change in percentage overweight for comparable time periods as performed on the combined experimental (treatment plus dropout) versus the control population indicates that the experimental group, even including those who dropped out, greatly outperformed the control population ($t = 2.95$, $p < 0.001$).

Matched Pairs

Valid comparisons of treatment and control group performance necessitated comparable treatment durations, ages, and percentage overweights. A matched set of 11 pairs of control and experimental patients was generated having closely similar characteristics. The mean percentage overweights, as seen in Table 12.2, reflect this pair-wise equivalence. The percentage overweight for a control child was computed over the actual treatment duration of his/her treated mate, using data from standard office visits. The matched pairs were selected randomly from the 14 treatment children, regardless of success or failure. The only criterion was our ability to find a comparable matched control child. A Wilcoxon matched-pairs signed ranks test on the change of percentage overweight over the treatment interval showed a striking improvement in the treated as opposed to the control patients (t = 3.0, $p < 0.005$—one-tail test).

Those who remained in treatment also outperformed those who dropped out. With measurement intervals of 7.6 months for dropout patients and 7.3 months for treatment children, a randomization test for two independent samples showed a larger group change in percentage overweight for the treatment condition (t = 2.49, $p < 0.025$). It should be noted that some of the dropout patients continued to improve without taking active part in the program. This might reflect the major impact of a relatively minor amount of intervention. Particularly in view of the rather consistent pattern of results seen in the control group, with either static or increasing levels of obesity, it would appear likely that a relatively modest intervention is effective for some children.

Of the 6 children in the sample under 8 yr of age, only 1 failed to make progress. Three of the four treatment failures were 9 yr of age or older. The mean percentage overweight of those who failed was initially 39%, which is very similar to the 43% overweight of the successes, but the failure tended towards the extremes of the distribution range.

DISCUSSION

The program results, as far as they are available, indicate that many moderately obese children can achieve a weight closer to their correct weight using a behaviorally oriented approach, at least over a period of active intervention. The reduction of obesity demonstrated in this program involves a gradual long-term adjustment, rather than a dramatic loss. The adjustment of eating behavior which was sought was of a permanent nature, congruent with the family's eating situation as it existed, rather than a program in which the eating situation was temporarily adapted to a prescribed diet plan. This approach involves an evolutionary adjustment, rather than a dramatic break with the past. Such an adjustment would seem particularly advantageous for the growing organism, where the growth process must proceed and where the child's eating occurs in the larger context of the family eating pattern.

The treatment results are very encouraging for those patients who remained in treatment. For those who did not, some made progress without the supervision of the program. It would appear, regarding these patients, that it is sufficient to acquaint them (and their mothers) with their difficulty and provide a preliminary analysis of its behavioral concordants. This phenomenon of dropout success has not been previously noted in such programs.

Factors associated with relative program success need to be separated into those related to continuation in the treatment and those related to success of treatment. There are substantial indications that these two facets of ultimate program success involve separate patient characteristics. One needs first to consider the characteristics of individuals who remain in treatment and then the factors related to success. Patients dropping the program appeared to be either the least or the most obese in the sample, their intake records were kept less well than those in treatment, and they were more likely to be males. There are indications that these subjects are generally younger and less likely to have normal weight parents. All of these factors are consistent with an interpretation of motivational problems in the drop-out patients, with separate etiologies for the most and least obese.

While the results of this study must certainly be considered preliminary, since only a long-term follow-up will enable us to judge its ultimate success, it is important to note that the kind of intervention described here is possible within the context of regular pediatric care, and hence can be long-term in nature. It should also be evident that the treated children currently have a substantial advantage over their untreated counterparts—an advantage which any long-term evaluation must compare not only to an ideal weight, but to the actual weight of untreated obese juveniles.

REFERENCES

Asher P. (1966) Fat babies and fat children: The prognosis of obesity in the very young, *Arch. Dis. Child. 41*, 672-673.

Christakis G., Sajecki S., Hillman R. W., Miller E., Blumenthal S., and Archer M. (1966) Effect of a combined nutrition education and physical fitness program on the weight status of obese high school boys, *Proceedings 25*, 15-19.

Knittle J. L. (1971) Childhood obesity, *Bull. N.Y. Acad. Med. 47*, 6, 579-589.

Lloyd J. K., Wolff O. H., and Whelen W. S. (1961) Childhood obesity: Long-term study of height and weight, *Brit. Med. J. 2*, 145-147.

Mayer J. (1968) *Overweight: Causes, Cost, and Control*, Prentice-Hall, Englewood Cliffs, N.J.

National Center for Health Statistics. (1970) *Height, Weight of Children in the United States, India, and the United Arab Republic Vital and Health Statistics*, No. 1000, Series 3 - No. 14, USD-HEW, U.S. Government Printing Office.

Parizkova J. et al. (1962) A study of changes in some functional indicators following reduction of excessive fat in obese children, *Physiologia Bohemoslovenia II*, 351-357.

Pekos D. S. (1960) Program and results of a camp for obese adolescent girls, *Postgraduate Med. 27*, 527-533.

Rohrbacher R. (1973) Influences of a special campus program for obese boys on weight loss, self concept, and body image, *Res. Quart. 44*, 150-157

Stuart R. B. and Davis B. (1972) *Slim Chance in a Fat World*, Research Press, Champaign, Ill.

Wolff O. H. (1955) Obesity in childhood, *Q. J. Med. 24*, 109.

AN INTEGRATED TREATMENT PROGRAM
FOR ANOREXIA NERVOSA

Ronald Leibman
Salvador Minuchin
Lester Baker

Summary: The use of behavior conditioning within the context of structural family therapy has proved effective in the treatment of anorexia nervosa. During the inpatient phase, a behavioral paradigm made access to physical activity dependent on weight gain; in the outpatient phase, social activities on the weekend were made dependent on weight gain. The authors found that early direct involvement of the family promotes significant rapid weight gain, while continued involvement of the family in therapy during the outpatient phase facilitates the necessary restructuring of the family to prevent relapses.

Reprinted from *American Journal of Psychiatry*, 1974, *131*, 432-436. Copyright 1974 by the American Psychiatric Association. Reprinted by permission.

Ronald Liebman and Salvador Minuchin are with the Philadelphia Child Guidance Clinic, 1700 Bainbridge St., Philadelphia, Pa. 19146, where Liebman is associate director of training, Division of Child Psychiatry, and Minuchin is director. Lester Baker is director, Clinical Research Center, Children's Hospital of Pennsylvania. The authors are also with the University of Pennsylvania School of Medicine, where Liebman is assistant professor of child psychiatry, Minuchin is professor of child psychiatry and pediatrics, and Baker is associate professor of pediatrics.

This paper won the 1973 Kenneth Appel Award of the Philadelphia County Medical Society and the 1973 Freda London Award of the American Association of Psychiatric Services for Children.

This work was supported in part by Public Health Service grants MH-21336 from the National Institute of Mental Health and RR-240 from the Research Resources Division of the National Institutes of Health.

The authors wish to thank Braullo Montalvo of the Philadelphia Child Guidance Clinic for his valuable assistance in the analysis of the family lunch sessions and in the organization and assignment of the family tasks, and B. Rosman and F. Hitchcock for their help in the preparation of the final manuscript.

Anorexia nervosa is defined as a clinical syndrome characterized by a voluntary refusal to eat, usually explained by the patient saying that he or she doesn't feel hungry, and a loss of 20 percent or more of the body weight without organic cause. It occurs more frequently in females, especially during adolescence and young adulthood. Cessation of menstruation and the clinical characteristics described by Hilde Bruch (disturbances of body image, misperception of internal physiological stimuli, a sense of ineffectiveness, and hyperactivity), although usually present, are not considered necessary for making the diagnosis. Other primary psychiatric diagnoses, such as depressive reactions, phobic states, and psychoses, must be ruled out.

Much has been written about the treatment of anorexia nervosa. Most investigators recommend hospitalization for a period ranging from several weeks to several months. Treatment has been focused on weight gain in the hospital and many methods have been used to achieve this (1). A combination of behavior therapy and chemotherapy has gained popularity for the treatment of the acute cachectic phase (2-5).

Little has been reported about the clinical course of anorectic patients after they leave the hospital. It would appear, however, that in many cases improvement is not sustained after they return to their home environments. Bruch (6) reported that 30 out of 50 patients for whom follow-up information was available were leading restricted lives, were institutionalized, had died of anorexia, or were still anorectic. Brady and Rieger (7) followed up 16 patients with anorexia (all of whom gained weight in the hospital); they reported two deaths, four rehospitalizations, and three cases of poor social adjustment at follow-up. Blinder, Freeman, and Stunkard (1), who were able to produce an average weight gain of 3.9 to 4.8 pounds per week in three hospitalized patients, reported that one of their patients committed suicide following discharge from the hospital after having a disturbing telephone conversation with her mother.

It is our contention that anorexia nervosa can best be approached with a therapeutic focus on the context of the patient's family. Direct involvement of the family early in the course of the acute cachectic phase promotes rapid, significant weight gain, facilitating the return of the patient to the family and peer group in a comparatively short period of time (two to three weeks). Continued involvement of the family in ongoing outpatient therapy makes it possible to restructure the family and thus to prevent relapses. Paradoxically, although investigators of anorexia have consistently described prominent family psychopathology (6, 8-10), few attempts have been made to modify the family environment to which the patient must return after discharge from the hospital.

For example, Reinhart and associates (11) reported on the outpatient management of 32 children with anorexia nervosa. Brief periods of hospitalization were used intermittently to separate the child from a family environment described as chaotic. But different therapists were used for the child and the parents and there was no collaboration between the child psychiatrist and the pediatric staff. Only Minuchin and associates (12-16) have reported on direct confrontation of a family's habitual interactional patterns to alleviate the symptoms of anorexia nervosa. Barcai (17) has also reported on the use of Minuchin's approach with two anorectic patients in Israel. The four patients reported in this paper were treated with a combination of operant conditioning and structural family therapy.

The four patients were all girls from white middle-class families. Medical evaluation revealed no organic etiology for the anorexia and weight loss. Their ages at the onset of symptoms ranged from nine years to 15 years, with an average of 12.6 years. The duration of symptoms prior to referral ranged from two months to nine months, with an average of 5.0 months. Prior to referral, two of the patients had had individually oriented psychotherapy and had been hospitalized for medical evaluation and weight gain, but they continued to lose weight. Weight loss ranged from 26 percent to 36 percent of total body weight, with an average of 31.7 percent at the time of referral.

THE TREATMENT PROGRAM

The integrated program has a series of phases with specific goals:

1. Admission to the Children's Hospital of Philadelphia for medical evaluation and weight gain.

2. Informal lunch sessions with the patient to assess the degree of negativism and anorexia.

3. Application of an operant reinforcement paradigm to initiate weight gain.

4. Family therapy lunch sessions to accelerate and reinforce weight gain.

5. Discharge from the hospital.

6. Application of an outpatient operant reinforcement paradigm as a family task to prevent weight loss.

7. Outpatient family therapy to change the structure and functioning of the family.

Inpatient Phase

After a complete medical and neurological evaluation failed to reveal the presence of an organic etiology for the weight loss, each of the patients was admitted to the Clinical Research Center of the Children's Hospital of Philadelphia. Periodically, the therapist ate lunch with the patient. On these occasions he told her that when he was hungry, his stomach hurt and he felt light-headed. He said that it felt good to eat and be satiated. No attempt was made to get the patient to eat her lunch. The therapist asked her permission to eat some small part of her food, such as a piece of carrot or celery. Then he offered to share part of his lunch with her. This procedure enabled the therapist to ascertain the degree of negativism and anorexia manifested by the patient. It also provided an opportunity to relate to her on the issues of sharing and eating food, thus avoiding a power struggle over the act of eating. During the lunch sessions, information regarding the patient's family, peer group, and school relationships was obtained in an informal fashion.

On the second day of hospitalization, the pediatrician explained the details of the operant reinforcement paradigm to the patient. On the third day, it was put into effect by the pediatrician and his nursing staff under the supervision of the family psychiatrist.* The behavior paradigm made access to physical activity completely contingent on weight gain (1). The patient was weighed every morning before breakfast. If she had gained less than half a pound over the previous morning's weight, she was not allowed out of bed for any reason. If she gained at least half a pound, she was allowed to be out of bed to eat, watch television, have visitors, and use the bathroom. She was also given a four to six-hour period of unrestricted activity on the ward or in the hospital.

The patient was allowed to discuss the details of her menu with the pediatrician, nurses, and dietitian. She could add or subtract certain foods as long as she ate a balanced diet at each meal. She could have three regular meals or five to six smaller ones. Confrontations over eating were avoided.

The pediatrician emphasized that the patient's family had nothing to do with the program in the hospital. All negotiations were between the patient and the staff. The pediatrician met with the patient's family, explained the program, and instructed them not to discuss it with the patient. Any questions were to be directed to him. The goal was to give the patient an increased sense of autonomy and responsibility for her physical state.

After the initiation of the inpatient behavior paradigm, there was in each case an initial period of slow weight gain. This decreased the anxiety of the staff and the patient's family, inspiring a more optimistic attitude. It also facilitated reaching the goals of the family therapy lunch sessions.

The family therapy lunch session was usually held at the end of the first week and included the patient, her parents and siblings, the pediatrician, and the family psychiatrist. This was the first time that the family met the psychiatrist and it marked the beginning of the transition from the inpatient

---

*The Clinical Research Center is a medical unit that in no way resembles a psychiatric hospital unit. In treating children with anorexia nervosa (or other psychosomatic illnesses) there is close collaboration between the family therapists and pediatricians. The nurses and other personnel are trained not to get into power struggles over the act of eating.

phase to the outpatient phase. It also demonstrated that the family psychiatrist and the pediatrician worked together in a mutually supportive way with the common goal of helping the patient and her family.

The goals of the family therapy lunch sessions are:

1. To enable the patient to eat in the presence of her parents without the development of a power struggle; this provides an entirely new experience for them with respect to eating. In our experience, it is necessary to make eating a private issue between the patient and the therapist in order to prevent self-defeating intrusions from the parents.

2. To redefine the presenting problem and dismantle the family's myth that they are fine except for the presence of their medically sick child. This formulation, which forces the patient into the rigid role of being the sole repository of all of the family's problems, has to be transformed into a recognition of the interpersonal transactional conflicts that exist between the parents and the patient. This will decrease the patient's centrality and the manipulative power of her symptoms.

At the end of the first lunch session, a weight goal was established for discharge. In the four cases discussed here, the process of weight gain was significantly accelerated by the lunch sessions. Each of the four patients was discharged from the hospital within seven to 14 days after the first lunch session. On the day of discharge, a second family lunch session was held to explain the goals of the outpatient program.

Outpatient Phase

In the outpatient phase, the family psychiatrist assumed the primary responsibility, with the pediatrician functioning in a supportive-consultative way. This was the reverse of the system used during the inpatient phase. The general goals of the outpatient phase are:

1. To eliminate the symptom of refusing to eat and to stimulate progressive weight gain. This has top priority. If the patient loses weight, the family will continue to concentrate on her symptoms as a way of avoiding or detouring family conflicts.

2. To elucidate the dysfunctional patterns in the family that reinforce the patient's symptoms.

3. To change the structure and functioning of the family system in order to prevent a recurrence of the symptoms or the development of a new symptom bearer. Weight gain alone is never considered sufficient. It is only a first step and must be followed by a restructuring of the family system.

The initial weight gain and family lunch sessions started the process of disengaging the patient from her role in the family's dysfunctional transactions. This process was continued by the assignment of an outpatient operant reinforcement paradigm, which the parents were to enforce. The behavior paradigm provided the parents with something concrete to do at home, which decreased their anxiety and previous feelings of helplessness in dealing with their sick child. The parents were supported in the endeavor by the psychiatrist and the pediatrician.

The outpatient paradigm was defined as an interpersonal process. The parents were told that it was their responsibility as parents to enforce the paradigm, and that if they were working together in a mutually supportive way they would be successful. If the patient refused to eat and lost weight, this would indicate that the parents were not working together. The patient was told that it was her responsibility to herself and to her parents to follow the paradigm. The authority for the paradigm rested with the psychiatrist and the pediatrician; if there was a crisis, the parents could call the therapist, but they were not to acquiesce to the patient's refusal to eat. This formulation also gave the patient increased responsibility and autonomy. As long as she followed the paradigm, she could have control over the entire area of eating.

The patient was told that she had to gain a minimum of two pounds a week in order to maintain normal activities. If she gained less than two pounds, from Friday to Friday, she was not allowed out of the house during the weekend and she could not have friends come to the house. In addition, a member of the family had to stay at home with her. This produced a great deal of stress in the family system, causing the members of the family to join together to ensure that the patient ate. If the patient gained between two and 2.5 pounds, she was allowed to be active on either Saturday or Sunday, but not both days. She was given the choice of days and the choice of activities. If she gained more than 2.5 pounds, she was allowed to be active on Friday night, Saturday, and Sunday.

Once weight gain was progressing in a gradual fashion, the outpatient family therapy was organized by the assignment of family tasks aimed at different subsystems of the family. The tasks were developed from an understanding of the individual, interpersonal, and family system dynamics. They were aimed at expediting changes in the structure, organization, and functioning of the family and at changing the quality of the interpersonal relationships in the family.

RESULTS OF THE TREATMENT PROGRAM

After the initiation of the behavior paradigm in the hospital, there was an initial lag period of about two or four days during which each of the patients was observed to be testing the staff members to see whether they were going to enforce the behavior paradigm. After the patient saw that the staff was consistently and persistently attending to the details of the program, there was an initial period of slow weight gain. Following the first family therapy lunch session, there was a period of much more rapid weight gain than had occurred with the use of the behavior paradigm alone. Seven to ten days after the first family lunch session, the patients were able to reach the weight goal required for discharge. After the weight gain and first family lunch session, there was a dramatic change in the affect and behavior of the patients. Manifestations of depression and negativism decreased significantly. They were able to choose their own meals and eat with other members of the hospital staff or their families in the cafeteria. In addition, the patients stated that they were too thin, that they needed to gain weight, and that the dieting and weight loss had occurred after an episode of emotional upset related to conflicts at home, at school, or in their peer groups. After the patient reached the goal required for discharge, a second family lunch session was held in order to ensure that the patient was still able to eat in the presence of her family. In addition, the date of discharge was announced and the details of the outpatient behavior paradigm were explained to the parents and the patient as a family task.

There was a two- or three-week period of testing at the beginning of the outpatient phase during which the patients did not gain the required two pounds. The psychiatrist and pediatrician supported the parents in enforcing the behavior paradigm. Then the patients began to gain the required amount of weight on a progressive weekly basis. The behavior paradigm was discontinued after the patient began to gain weight on a consistent basis or when the patient reached the goal determined by the pediatrician.

In all four cases, as weight gain continued the focus shifted from eating and the behavior paradigm to concern about interpersonal issues. As intrafamilial and interpersonal issues began to be resolved, the emphasis shifted to school and community activities and the peer group relationships. Within the family, there was a gradual shifting of emphasis to the parental dyad. At this point, the parents were seen separately, with periodic family sessions as needed. Occasionally the children were seen alone to discuss age-appropriate issues. The general goal was the gradual disengagement of the children from the conflicts between their parents and their movement into age-appropriate peer group activities.

In summary, the length of hospitalizations varied from eight to 21 days, with an average of 14.5 days. Weight gain in the hospital varied from one-third to one-half the amount of weight lost prior to referral. The treatment modalities used were the operant reinforcement paradigms and family therapy as described above. Medications were *not* used in any of the cases. The duration of family therapy ranged from four months to ten months, with an average of 7.2 months. All of the patients were able to reach and maintain normal weight with the restoration of normal eating patterns.

DISCUSSION AND CONCLUSIONS

It is beyond the scope of this paper to discuss the theoretical foundations of structural family therapy and the relationship between family structure and a child's psychosomatic symptoms (12-16). The four families were each characterized by weak generational boundaries; ineffective, divided parents; and little autonomy and privacy for individual members. They were rigid systems and were incapable of resolving conflicts, finding solutions to problems, or dealing effectively with stressful, frustrating situations.

By concentrating only on the symptoms of the patient, the parents were able to deny and avoid dealing with problems that existed between them or with the siblings. The symptoms were therefore reinforced within the context of the family. When the structure of the family had been changed, family and parental conflicts could be resolved. Then it was possible for the patient to move in the direction of increased peer group activities and relationships. If the structure of the family is not changed, continuation or reappearance of the patient's symptoms (or the appearance of a new symptom bearer) can be expected.

In summary, with a clinical disorder that has a significant mortality rate (five to 15 percent), the physician's top priority is to ensure the survival of the patient. The behavior paradigm and the family lunch sessions in the hospital begin the processes of weight gain and of disengaging the patient from the arena of submerged parental conflicts. The outpatient behavior paradigm and the family tasks continue to support weight gain and to decrease the patient's role as a means of detouring family conflicts. When used in the context of structural family therapy, behavior modification paradigms are effective methods of avoiding self-defeating power struggles.

It will be noted that phenothiazines and antidepressants were not used in the acute cachectic phase. However, psychotropic drugs could be used, as were the behavior paradigms, as a lever to start the therapeutic process moving. The family interventions, such as the lunch sessions and the family tasks, are vital to the outcome of therapy. Other therapeutic modalities will be undermined unless there are constructive changes in the family system that make it possible for the family to prevent relapses and to support the continued growth and development of its members.

REFERENCES

1. Blinder BJ, Freeman DM, Stunkard AJ: Behavior therapy of anorexia nervosa. *Am J Psychiatry 126*:1093-1098, 1970.

2. Crisp AH: Clinical and therapeutic aspects of anorexia. *J Psychosom Res* 9:67-78, 1965.
3. Dally P, Sargant W. A new treatment of anorexia. *Br Med J* 1:1770-1773, 1960.
4. Dally P, Sargant W: A treatment and outcome of anorexia. *Br Med J 2*: 293-295, 1966
5. Stunkard AJ: New therapies for the eating disorders. *Arch Gen Psychiatry 26*:391-398, 1972.
6. Bruch H: *Eating Disorders.* New York, Basic Books, 1973
7. Brady JP, Rieger W: Behavioral treatment of anorexia nervosa. Read at the International Symposium on Behavior Modification, Minneapolis, Minn, Oct 4-6, 1972.
8. Selvini-Palazzoli M: The families of patients with anorexia nervosa, in *The Child and His Family.* Edited by Anthony I, Koupernik C. New York, John Wiley & Sons, 1970, pp 319-332.
9. Tolstrup K: The necessity for differentiating eating disorders, *Ibid*, pp 311-317.
10. Shafii M, Salguero C, Finch S: Anorexia adieu: psychopathology and treatment of anorexia nervosa in latency-age siblings. Read at the annual meeting of the American Academy of Child Psychiatry, New Orleans, La, Oct 12-15, 1972.
11. Reinhart JB, Kenna MD, Succop RA: Anorexia nervosa in children: outpatient management. *J Child Psychiatry 11*:114-131, 1972
12. Minuchin S: The use of an ecological framework in the treatment of a child, in *The Child and His Family*, Edited by Anthony I, Koupernik C. New York, John Wiley & Sons, 1970, pp 41-57.
13. Minuchin S: Anorexia nervosa: interaction around the family table. Read at the Institute for Juvenile Research, Chicago, Ill, Jan 8, 1971
14. Minuchin S: *Families & Family Therapy.* Cambridge, Mass, Harvard University Press, 1974.
15. Minuchin S, Baker L, Rosman B, et al: Psychosomatic illness in children: a new conceptual model. Philadelphia, Philadelphia Child Guidance Clinic, 1973 (unpublished)
16. Minuchin S, Baker L, Liebman R, et al: Anorexia nervosa; successful application of a family therapy approach (abstract). *Pediatr Res 7*:294, 1973.
17. Barcai A: Family therapy in the treatment of anorexia nervosa. *Am J Psychiatry 128*:286-290, 1971.

INDEX

ABOUT THE EDITORS

Dr. Ben J. Williams is an Assistant Professor in the Department of Psychiatry at Baylor College of Medicine and is Chief Child Psychologist in the Child and Adolescent Psychiatry Clinic at Texas Children's Hospital. He is responsible for the training of clinical psychology post doctoral and intern level personnel as well as practicum students in clinical child psychology. Dr. Williams has a private psychotherapy practice with children and adults. He is also past president and co-founder of the Houston Behavioral Therapy Association (HBTA).

Dr. Williams did his graduate studies at the University of Tennessee, completing an internship in the Department of Psychiatry at North Carolina Memorial Hospital and was post doctoral fellow in the Division for Disorders of Development and Learning in the Child Development Institute at the University of North Carolina. Dr. Williams' interests lie in the area of behavioral medicine, the hyperactive child and his parents as well as familiar hypertension. He is currently involved in research on the hyperactive child in the classroom and on the role of familiar hypertension in children. He has published in the area of hyperactivity, obesity and familiar hypertension.

Dr. John P. Foreyt is an Associate Professor in the Departments of Medicine and Psychiatry at Baylor College of Medicine. In addition to teaching and consulting, Dr. Foreyt serves as principal investigator of the Baylor College of Medicine National Heart and Blood Vessel Research and Demonstration Center's Diet Modification Clinic.

Dr. Foreyt has published widely in the area of behavioral treatments of obesity and dietary behavior, behavior modification techniques in institutions, cognitive behavior therapy, and psychological assessment. Before coming to Baylor, Dr. Foreyt was a faculty member at Florida State University and Director of the Behavior Modification Taken Economy Program at Florida State Hospital, Chattahoochee. He received his Ph.D. in clinical psychology from Florida State University in 1969.

Dr. Ken Goodrick received his Ph.D. in psychology from the University of Houston in 1975. He is currently researching health behavior modification, and his private practice deals with obesity treatment. He has worked with learning disabled, retarded and autistic children as a behavior therapist, and has taught child psychology and adolescent development at the university level. He is also a consultant to Baylor College of Medicine and the American Heart Association in the area of developing health education curricula for school children.